A Life That Matters

D1301913

A Life That Matters

Transforming Faces,
Renewing Lives

KENNETH E. SALYER, MD

CENTER
STREET

NEW YORK   BOSTON   NASHVILLE

Center Street
Hachette Book Group
237 Park Avenue
New York, NY 10017

www.CenterStreet.com

Printed in the United States of America

RRD-C

First edition: June 2013
10 9 8 7 6 5 4 3 2 1

Center Street is a division of Hachette Book Group, Inc.
The Center Street name and logo are trademarks of
Hachette Book Group, Inc.

The Hachette Speakers Bureau provides a wide range of authors for speaking events. To find out more, go to www.HachetteSpeakersBureau.com or call (866) 376-6591.

The publisher is not responsible for websites (or their content) that are not owned by the publisher.

Library of Congress Cataloging-in-Publication Data

Salyer, Kenneth E.
    A life that matters : transforming faces, renewing lives / Kenneth Salyer.—1st ed.
        p. ; cm.
    ISBN 978-1-4555-1512-7 (trade pbk.)—ISBN 978-1-4555-1513-4 (ebook)
    I. Title.
    [DNLM: 1. Salyer, Kenneth E. 2. Craniofacial Abnormalities—surgery—Autobiography. 3. Surgery, Plastic—Autobiography. 4. Child. 5. History, 20th Century. 6. History, 21st Century. WZ 100]

    617.95092—dc23
    [B]
                                                            2012041842

For my family,
my wife, Luci;
my children, Ken and Leigh;
and my grandchildren, Ken III, Hart VI, Ashley, Everett,
Thomas, and Adelle.

I will not die an unlived life.
I will not live in fear
Of falling or catching fire.
I choose to inhabit my days,
To allow my living to open me,
To make me less afraid,
More accessible;
To loosen my heart
Until it becomes a wing,
A torch, a promise.
I choose to risk my significance,
To live so that which came to me as seed
Goes to the next as blossom,
And that which came to me as blossom,
Goes on as fruit.

Dawna Markova

Contents

A Life That Matters

A Life That Matters

Gabriela Morales was beautiful—or at least I could imagine how beautiful she could become. Gabriela had been born to a poor Mexican family, and her early life had been terribly compromised by a congenital malformation of her face that led many to turn away from her, cruelly taunt her, even presume she was possessed by evil spirits.

Gabriela, now sixteen, was raised in a shantytown in Tijuana and had been introduced to the staff of the World Craniofacial Foundation, an organization I established in 1989, by an American mission worker. Noting her abnormally wide-set eyes and dramatically malformed nose—which had been made even more unsightly by a well-meaning but untrained physician soon after she was born—the missionary imagined that with our help, the very shy girl with big dreams could, in fact, fulfill them one day.

At home in Dallas, when I read reports and saw photographs of Gabi, I was quickly sure that one day she could have a normal face—a birthright I believe all the world's children possess. The foundation raised funds to send her and her parents to Mexico City, where surgeons at an extraordinary reconstructive plastic surgery and teaching center—established three decades ago by my dear friend and colleague Dr. Fernando Ortiz Monasterio—could transform Gabi's face and set her young life on a very hopeful new course. And when I met dark-eyed and engaging Gabriela in person on a bright April morning in Mexico's capital city, I was certain that she, like thousands of other patients I've met during my five-decade career, had a bright future indeed.

The Hospital General Dr. Manuel Gea González, located in Mexico City's frenetic Tlalpan district, is surrounded by a high metal-barred fence, its entrances guarded by policemen carrying automatic weapons. On any day, literally thousands of impoverished Mexicans wait patiently for services, often for many hours, yet early every Tuesday morning, the hospital's plastic and reconstructive surgery unit becomes what its recently deceased founder called "the most exciting clinic in the world, the only place I want to be"—a clinic where young patients like Gabi come from throughout the country to be evaluated by a team comprising some of the finest craniofacial surgeons in the world.

In my travels around the globe, performing surgeries and helping establish surgical centers in countries where top-quality medicine is seldom practiced, it is clinics like this one that demonstrate to me that even the very poor *can* receive excellent medical care at costs that don't bankrupt health-care systems. And with every passing day, I believe more strongly that Gabriela and everyone like her *can* be offered the basic human right of a normal face.

Consider what life entails for children like Gabi before they are treated; imagine the constant rejection and soul-killing ridicule and the virtual impossibility of succeeding in school, making friends, or one day falling in love. For many centuries, people with facial deformities were locked away, and oftentimes, infants with terrible deformities were simply not allowed to live. And still all too often today, people with shocking facial abnormalities are shunned, hidden, shamed, and tormented.

I've believed passionately since I was a young surgeon in Dallas in the early 1960s that all the world's children deserve to lead normal lives, yet for one child in every five hundred, a normal life is impossible without craniofacial surgery. Forty years ago, medicine offered little hope to patients with severe deformities of the skull, jaw, and face, but in pioneering new surgical protocols that once were unimaginable, it's been my goal—and my life's great joy—to help profoundly change the outlook for these patients and their families. What once was impossible is now a practical reality because of the advancements of modern medical technology and the extraordinarily well-honed skills of a host of professionals.

A craniofacial surgeon never operates alone. He or she serves as both surgeon and impresario, performing incredibly intricate surgical techniques as well as coordinating the work of a highly skilled interdisciplinary team in which each member is absolutely essential to a positive patient outcome. Pediatric neurosurgeons, pediatric anesthesiologists, neuroradiologists, pediatric intensivists, neuro-ophthalmologists, pediatric ophthalmologists, otolaryngologists, orthodontists, speech pathologists, geneticists, anthropologists, pedodontists, pediatric nurses, psychologists, and social workers play vitally important supporting roles, and developing and coordinating a cadre of exceptional professionals can sometimes pose many complexities.

My patient Michael Hatfield, for example, was born with eyes on the sides of his head and without a nose. As a young boy, Michael was shocking to look at, and his mother reported that "people assume he's retarded, incapable of interaction or emotion, just one of nature's rejects." Without a series of complex surgeries, Michael's life would be effectively over as it began.

By the time he was eighteen, I had operated on Michael four times, creating new orbits for the eyes in the front of his skull, moving his eyes naturally close together, creating a nose whose structural base was a piece of his rib, and sculpting natural-looking cheeks, forehead, and ears. The surgeries were anything but simple, but Michael was always accepting, determined, and confident. He eventually became quite outgoing and vivacious, playing football and tennis and developing his natural leadership skills—and he and I became very close. Surgery on another patient prevented me from attending his high school graduation in Corpus Christi, Texas, but I was as proud as his parents were when he enrolled in Emory University in Atlanta, then returned to Texas to attend law school at the University of Houston. Today, Michael is married and the father of a six-month-old son, and he's creating a career focused on innovative ways for companies to maximize their employees' inherent potential. It's work Michael was made for, and it's hard for me to describe how full my heart is when I consider how rich his life has become—and how terribly at risk he was for having no life at all.

Ashley Ashcroft was born with what is called a cleft lip and palate. A portion of her upper lip, her palate, and the floor of her nose were missing, and her abilities to eat, breathe, smell, and talk were seriously compromised. Ashley *had* to have surgery to survive. But more than merely survive, I wanted her to *live* in ways that fulfilled her enormous potential. After seven surgeries over many years, Ashley emerged as a strong, fiercely intelligent, self-directed, and beautiful young woman. No longer limited in any way, Ashley attended college, then trained as a certified physician's assistant, and today she works in the ophthalmology department at MD Anderson Cancer Center in Houston. Ashley grew comfortable with and interested in the world of medicine during her many years as a patient, and like me, she discovered how wonderfully rewarding a life of caregiving can be. She, like Michael and hundreds more patients, has constantly reminded me over the years that young lives like theirs must *never* be sacrificed to their deformities, and that every one of us—young and old—deserves a face with which we can bravely meet the world.

Long ago, medicine intrigued me as a career because it would allow me to pursue science, help others, and explore the challenges of what couldn't yet be accomplished—but might be. Early in my training, I discovered that I was drawn to surgery; I considered many options and specialties, but ultimately only reconstructive plastic surgery truly captured my imagination at a time when even many major large-city hospitals lacked plastic surgery departments.

More than sixteen thousand surgeries and nearly fifty years later, I've been blessed not only to have helped transform thousands of patients' lives, but to have transformed my own as well. This work has given deep meaning to the totality of my life and has allowed me to discover my core sense of purpose—not just cutting, sawing, and suturing, but freeing the *spirits* of my patients, allowing them to look comfortably in the mirror and understand that they are not freaks but, in fact, are vitally important members of the human family.

Along the way, I've observed a striking phenomenon: many young people with terribly disfiguring diseases possess special gifts—insights, sensitivities, and a profound humanity that you commonly see only in people far older—gifts that aren't readily visible until you get to know them. People like Michael, Ashley, and Gabriela, who lack normal skulls, jaws, noses, or eyes, nonetheless express the courage to face what life brings that is rare in other patients I treat. Their buoyant personalities and resolute perseverance inspire and renew me and virtually everyone they encounter.

I've also come to know another kind of patient—victims of unspeakable violence whose faces have been destroyed by evildoers—and my heart breaks for them. I've met a number of women in Uganda, for example, whose noses and ears were cut off by enemies as a wicked blood sport. And the morning I met Gabriela in Mexico City, I also met Magdalena Ayala, a twenty-two-year-old Guatemalan woman whose husband had horrifically sliced off her nose, lips, and chin with a machete in a fit of rage. Like the Ugandan women, Magdalena seemed robbed of her soul. She was vacant eyed, empty, far removed from the world, and I tried to understand that perhaps that is the only response possible when your face is taken from you.

The sole light in Magdalena's life was that, with the help of the Guatemalan government, she had come to a hospital where her face and her soul could slowly be returned to her in a series of highly complex surgeries. But for years to come, she and those Ugandan women who had suffered similar attacks would reexperience that terrible violence every day of their lives—simply by looking in the mirror.

Whether they are victims of violence or of accidents or were born with disfiguring congenital disorders, I've been struck by how often my patients become dedicated to helping others with similar challenges—volunteering in clinics, doggedly raising funds for research, assisting individual patients and their families, speaking publicly to raise awareness of the worldwide need for help, even pursuing medical careers in craniofacial surgery or related specialties.

Like those of us who work in this field, craniofacial patients—and those who once were—remain particularly sensitive throughout their lives to the truth that each person deserves not just to exist but to thrive. In valuing individual lives and striving to make them better, we value all of humanity.

Sixteen-year-old Gabriela, who soon would undergo the first of several surgeries, and whose face would one day become one she was proud of, reminded me of the time long ago when I was her age. Growing up in Kansas, I suffered from asthma from the time I was very young, struggling to breathe, often requiring oxygen, and I vividly remember hearing my parents discuss with doctors the possibility that I might die. As I reached my early teens, I remained isolated from schoolmates, housebound, lonely, and awkward, just as Gabriela was, and I couldn't imagine becoming an adult, let alone one who might live a valuable life.

But I eventually grew healthy enough that in a few years I

began to work as an intern in my father's dentistry practice and dared imagine the possibility that I could become a physician. I began to drive myself toward that end, becoming absolutely single-minded, even obsessed with my personal pursuit of excellence. In college, I demanded the very best of myself and was often the last person to leave labs and study groups, reading late into every night, ensuring that my grades were always very high and ultimately graduating from medical school in the top tenth of my class. As a young surgeon, I intensified an already unflinching dedication to hard work and extremely high standards, and I owe my career accomplishments not to superior intellect, talent, or luck, but to two other attributes that shape the totality of who I am.

The first is a deep desire never to fail. That drive has made me a fine surgeon, I know, and has helped me play a seminal role I'm proud of in the development of craniofacial surgery. In operating rooms, thousands of times, it's been a critical ally as I've painstakingly lifted young faces away from terribly misshapen skulls, then reshaped those skulls with complex instruments, simple scalpels, and saws, as well as with my fingertips and hands. Each time I've created a new skull, nose, ear, or chin for an unfortunate child, or for one of the thousands of adults who've been my patients, I've been blessed by my compulsion to do my work extremely well.

The second attribute that has served me successfully is a strong and emotional compassion—rooted in my childhood, I'm sure—for youngsters whose deformities destroy their opportunities to *live*. I ache for them; my life is richest when I'm able to help them, and my great cause is encouraging people everywhere to open their hearts and recognize that possessing a face you aren't forced to hide is a fundamental human right—as important to a fully lived life as freedom from fear or want.

As I reach my midseventies, that pursuit of excellence, that compassion—and a *passion* for this work that still helps me spring out of bed each morning—continue to grow. I'm very optimistic about the progress we're making in the developed world in bringing treatment to everyone who needs it. But in developing countries, much remains to be accomplished, and I devote the majority of my time to sounding a clarion call not just for understanding but for *action*. The need is too great and the lives of children who possess tragic faces are too precious for me to simply sit by and wish them well. No one needs to become a craniofacial surgeon to offer assistance; there are hundreds of ways we all can bring awareness, funding, and vital work to this great cause. Your compassion and commitment, I can guarantee, will be met with the priceless knowledge that you have helped give young people faces, and thereby have given them the great gift of themselves.

When people possess normal faces—when they can see, hear, speak, and chew normally, and when they're not forced to hide their faces from the world—their spirits can soar, and nothing in life seems more important to me than that possibility, a hope that lifts each of us toward the best lives we can make.

Our faces are *us* in a very fundamental way. Four of our five senses are located in our faces and heads; it's with them that we encounter and understand the world around us. Just as importantly, with our faces we give those with whom we interact a vital glimpse of who we truly are. Our faces communicate—far more accurately and eloquently than does speaking, in many ways—what our minds believe and our hearts hold true. Imagine expressing love, for example, without a face behind which you're comfortable. Imagine the despair of ever receiving it.

On the pages that follow, you'll meet a number of the young people with heartbreaking craniofacial abnormalities whose challenges and boundless courage have stirred me to become a tireless advocate on their behalf. As the book unfolds, I recount not just my own journey but also the stories of children from around the world whose lives might otherwise have been lost, people who remain bright in memory and very dear to my heart.

I think of Lynn Beaver, the remarkable young woman with Crouzon's syndrome who, in 1974, was the first patient whose face and skull I resculpted and whose life was renewed in wonderful ways. I remember, too, Georgette Couvall, who was born in 1975, the obstetrician who attended her birth telling her father, "It's a girl, but I've never seen anything like her." Over the course of thirteen surgeries and many years, I was able to transform Georgette into a beautiful young woman, and she became a dear friend, someone who today works tirelessly in support of other craniofacial patients and on behalf of the World Craniofacial Foundation.

I can never forget ten-year-old Petero Byakatonda, a Ugandan boy who also suffered from Crouzon's. With the help of the foundation to which I continue to devote my energies, Petero was able to travel to Dallas for surgery, and

I remember him singing in his native Luganda as he was wheeled into surgery, "God, we have come in front of you. Please bless us and keep us."

My heart still aches for Romanian twin sisters Anastasia and Tatiana Dogaru, conjoined at the head, who shared far too many vital brain structures, as well as compromised hearts and kidneys, we discovered, for our surgical team to attempt to separate them. And I still marvel at the astonishing journey of Egyptian twins Mohamed and Ahmed Ibrahim, whom we did successfully separate in an extraordinarily complex procedure that we planned for more than a year and that lasted for thirty-six hours. A year later, in a second, groundbreaking operation performed on the now separated boys, we constructed new skulls for each of them—something unimaginable only a few years before—and today they are schoolboys thriving at home in Egypt.

The Ugandan women, robbed of ears, noses, and their very selves, will always haunt me, of course, as will Magdalena, the victim of her husband's unspeakable violence; and I'll always delight in my memory of Gabriela's bright and optimistic smile that day I met her in Mexico City, remembering that like her, I was once young and hopeful and determined to live a good life.

Gabi and thousands of children like her have been the focus of my work; they have given me countless rewards, and they continue to be my cause. The book you hold in your hands is a call to action—a call for us to do everything we can to help young people like Gabi fulfill the great promise of their lives. It's also a reminder to each of us to be inspired by how these young people have overcome terrible disfigurement and to transfer that awareness to our own lives, working to transform our own shortcomings, setbacks, and personal challenges into lives we continually renew for the better. Life *is* transformation, and in our own ways, each of us—like so many of my patients—can overcome any obstacle, no matter how great.

Chapter One

Sick and Afraid

What I remember most from my childhood is my fear of dying. I had asthma; I wheezed, struggled to breathe, and was constantly weak, spending much of my time in bed. My body was never going to be healthy, it seemed, let alone robust, and if I survived into adulthood, I'd have to make my way with my brain and not my brawn. Yet I wasn't at all sure I *would* grow up.

I was born in Kansas City, Kansas, on August 18, 1936. My mom and dad and I lived with my grandparents in a house at 711 Sandusky just off Seventh Street, a few blocks from downtown Kansas City. As early as I can remember, a heavy metal oxygen tank stood by my bed, and an oxygen mask attached to it helped me breathe. But breathing—simply breathing—was difficult, and it was frightening.

The Depression still raged, and we were poor. My grandfather Salyer drove a truck and helped support us while my father attended dental school; my mother worked at a five-and-dime on Minnesota Avenue and spent lots of time caring for her mother, my grandmother Warren—a tall, buxom, commanding woman who was a Cherokee and had lived her early years in Indian Territory in Oklahoma.

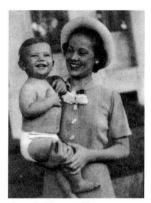

Dr. Salyer at three months with his mother, Laurene

Mom and Dad were dedicated to each other and showed love and affection throughout their entire marriage. They loved to dance, and my two sisters and I have lasting memories of them smiling and dancing. Our whole family danced together and played music as we were growing up. Both Mom and Dad were great role models when it came to giving back to the community—service to others was always a part of life at home.

One event of these years that may very well have influenced my choice of specialty occurred when, as a teenager, my younger sister, Sandra, was riding in a car with friends when a cherry bomb blew up in the backseat. She was in surgery all night but lost the sight in one eye. That memory and its effect on her as a young person stayed with me.

My mother was a strong presence—and distinct from my father, who was a quiet and gentle man. And although I knew he was every bit as concerned about my asthma as my mother was, she seemed to be in a constant state of alarm about whether I would survive the night. I picked up on her fears, of course, and they fed my own, as did hearing the doctor tell my mom and dad late one evening, "He's a trouper, and we're doing everything we can for him, but you've got to be prepared for the possibility that he won't survive."

Like many Americans in that era, most of my ancestors were immigrants from Europe. Three Salyer brothers came to the United States from France before the Civil War—two settled in New England, and the third became a slave-owning farmer in Kentucky. A village near his farm became known as Salyersville—and I was made its honorary mayor on my only visit decades later.

Eventually, my great-grandfather James Clinton Salyer made his way to Kansas, where he worked as a circuit-riding judge, as Lincoln had done. But the man evidently was no Lincoln; he was a hard drinker and terrible family man, and my grandfather B. A. Salyer was forced to go to work to support the family when he was only in the fourth grade. My grandfather labored in the fields for less than a dollar a day, never received any more education, and worked hard every day of his life, starting a canning company, selling pickles and wholesale fruits and vegetables. Granddad would wake up at two or three in the morning, hitch up his horse and buggy, go down to the local market, load up his goods, and peddle to stores in the area surrounding Topeka, Kansas. By the late 1910s, he had built a multimillion-dollar business, complete with a fleet of tractor-trailer trucks and several warehouses, and dozens of people worked for him.

He was a classic go-getter, and building his business and wealth were accomplishments he and his family were very proud of. But in the crash of 1929, he and the family lost

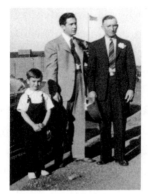

Dr. Salyer at age four with his grandfather Benjamin A. Salyer and his father, Everett

everything—everything except the single truck in which he subsequently made endless trips to Denver, where he would buy a load of vegetables and fruit he would sell to grocery stores along the route back home to eastern Kansas.

My maternal grandfather, George Warren, worked for the Union Pacific Railroad; I remember that sometimes he wore a pistol strapped to his hip, and I got to hunt with him a few times when I was well enough. I loved being around both men, as well as my two grandmothers. I felt very close to them and spent a lot of time with all four of them, particularly in the early years when my dad was consumed with the challenges and pressures of dental school and my mom was working full-time.

When my father graduated, he became the first professional in either the Salyer or the Warren family, and everyone took pride in his accomplishment. I attended the graduation ceremony as a two-year-old, I'm told, and my first memories of my dad are of someone everyone looked up to. He was a kind and always caring man, and people felt comfortable going to him for their dental work.

One of my dad's closest friends was a physician named Louis Gloyne; he was the fellow who delivered me, in fact, and his office was near my father's in a building in downtown Kansas City. Dr. Gloyne was both a family friend and the family physician, and beginning early in my life he was determined to see what he could do to improve my asthma and make me healthy. He treated me with sulfa drugs, tested me for every allergy under the sun, suggested particular diets, and recommended that I be kept indoors—and I know it troubled him that he couldn't simply cure me.

Kansas has four distinct seasons, including winters with plenty of snow, and hot summers when every weed imaginable grows wildly, and neither the doctor nor my parents could be sure ultimately whether I was terribly allergic to the mold that grew in the damp recesses of our house, or to ragweed or other summer pollens, or whether something else was at the root of my problems. They did accurately ascertain that I was violently allergic to cats—I still am—but simply keeping me away from cats wasn't enough to keep my bronchial airway open. With an overprotective mother looking after me, buttressed by a physician who was eager, too, to ensure that my condition didn't worsen, playing outdoors with other kids was simply out of the question.

It wasn't until the United States entered World War II and my father became an army dentist stationed at Fort Bliss in El Paso, Texas, that my sequestered life began to broaden. I certainly fared better in the dry desert air on the US-Mexico border; I had energy I'd never had before, and little by little, my parents allowed me to spend time outdoors. For the first time in my life, I began to play with other kids, to run and jump and swing, and I loved it. I'd reached the third grade, and suddenly dying didn't seem a certainty. Maybe I *could* grow up; maybe I could be normal.

My dad had been a tennis champion in his youth in Topeka, and he began to teach me the game during the eighteen months we spent in El Paso—something that would have been unthinkable just a year or so before. The rest of the world was consumed by a terrible war, but for me, that time in the desert was a glimpse of a life I'd feared I'd never have. In Texas, I wasn't forced to think of myself as being sick; for the first time, I thought of myself as *alive*.

Although my parents certainly celebrated my improvement, remaining in the desert Southwest wasn't an option when the war ended in 1945. Our extended family remained in and around Kansas City—and living near family was important to us—so we returned, and so did my wheezing and coughing and fighting for every breath. Yet by then I'd had a taste of life, of what it meant to venture outside the house, to play and interact with other kids and challenge myself physically. I still didn't have much confidence—and I was shaken by the dramatic return of my asthma—but I was different somehow.

I returned to Kansas with a newfound determination to be as normal as I could be. I spent lots of time by myself—listening to *The Green Hornet* and *The Lone Ranger* on the radio—but little by little, I developed friendships and grew physically stronger. And I spent far more time outdoors in Kansas than I ever had before, playing cowboys and Indians and other games with a growing circle of friends.

You would think that my long isolation and nearly constant solitude might have resulted in my becoming an excellent student—but that sadly wasn't the case. I was never a voracious reader; I didn't discover the world via books, and although I wasn't the worst student in school, As and Bs weren't my most common grades. I was a tall, skinny, awkward kid, and easy to make fun of—and more than a few bullies found taunting me irresistible. That might have been part of the reason school was never a place I was eager to be, but more than anything else, I know I was preoccupied with a fear of dying that somehow I couldn't shake.

Even well into junior high school, if I tried to shovel the sidewalk in front of our house, my airway would tighten, I'd begin to wheeze and fight for air, and I would panic. In the summer, the same thing repeatedly happened when I'd try to mow the lawn. I just couldn't do it—and I would have loved to. You can't imagine how great it would have felt—and how proud I would have been—if I'd simply been able to cut the grass. It was hard to envision ever being productive, ever lending a hand, ever being strong and capable. The bullies were right, I decided: I wasn't worth much. I was often in tearful despair.

By the time I reached high school, I'd grown stronger, at least a bit, and I'd begun to be a better student. I still struggled with writing, literature, and languages, but I discovered an interest in science and math—even some real aptitude in those areas. I didn't have any idea yet where those skills might lead me, but at least they were an aspect of me I could feel good about. Then, in a vocational studies class in my sophomore year, the teacher assigned us to write a report on a profession that interested us.

By that time, I'd become a bit of a regular at my dad's dental office—just hanging out at first, then doing a variety of jobs he trained me to do in his lab—and I remember that I loved to tag along when Dad and his good friend Dr. Gloyne got together, the two men letting me join them for a malted milk shake at the neighborhood drugstore often enough that I felt kind of like a colleague.

I'd been a regular patient of Dr. Gloyne's all my life, of course, and I thought I had a good sense of what it was like to be a family practitioner. So it made sense to write my assigned report about the life of a dentist or a physician. For some reason, I chose medicine—maybe because I worried that my teacher would think it was too easy if I chose to write about my father's profession.

Each of us in the class had to read our report aloud, and I doubt that mine was particularly impressive. Yet I brought an unmistakable enthusiasm to the subject; I made it sound as if being a doctor was a terrific thing, and that was the day my classmates nicknamed me Doc, a sobriquet that stuck with me throughout my high school career. I kind of liked the name, to be honest, and at least privately, I began direct-

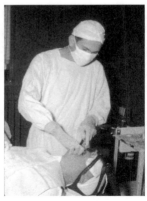

Dr. Salyer, in his teens, acting as his father's assistant in dental surgery

ing myself toward the possibility that one day I would *be* a doctor.

Although it was perhaps remote, the possibility that I had the stuff to become a doctor really motivated me to overcome my physical challenges as best I could and gain a bit of the self-confidence I'd never had. With the help of a few teachers who assured me that I could achieve whatever I set my mind to, I finally became the student I'd never been before. I couldn't play football or basketball—the sports that "mattered," as far as most of the kids in the school were concerned—but I worked hard at tennis, lettering in the sport in my junior and senior years, and I became a key member of a team that once won thirty-one straight matches. Because of my asthma, I always had trouble running up to the net, but my forehand and backhand strokes were sound, I had a good serve, and I pushed myself as hard as I could.

On and off the court, asthma still limited me—but by the time I turned sixteen it was a limitation rather than a disability, and I'd become normal enough in my junior year that I even managed to have developed a relationship with a girl, something that would have been unimaginable just a year or two before. Even when I contracted mononucleosis from her, I gamely endured the illness and my slow recovery as proof that I'd become a regular guy.

I was so thoroughly and proudly a Kansan that when it came time to decide where I would go to college, there really wasn't any decision to make. I attended the University of Kansas at nearby Lawrence with the hope that I would be accepted into the university's medical school as soon as I completed the institution's undergraduate science prerequi-sites. I was certain I wanted to be a doctor by now and was eager to get under way. But the medical school wanted its students to have a well-rounded undergraduate education, and each time I applied I was rejected—and told to complete my bachelor of science degree, *then* to apply.

I wasn't happy with having to wait, particularly because in addition to imagining a lifelong career as a physician, my college girlfriend, Shaaron Steeby, and I had made the decision to marry during my junior year at Lawrence. It was 1957 and neither of us had turned twenty-one yet; in retrospect, we were probably far too young to marry and begin to create a family, but we were in love. And there was something else, I'm sure: I wanted to leave the long and dif-ficult years of my childhood behind me; I wanted to dive into adulthood, and no doubt I imagined that marriage and children—and medical school—would be fast-track tickets out of my isolated and sickly life and into a world in which I was a full participant.

Because the University of Kansas School of Medicine turned me down, and perhaps a little impulsively, I decided to apply to the dental school at the University of Missouri–Kansas City instead. My father had led a successful and sat-isfying life as a dentist, after all, and the dental school was at home in Kansas City, and my parents and Shaaron were supportive. I was accepted, and my grades placed me in the top ten percent of my class at the end of my first year, but something was wrong. I couldn't escape the growing real-ization that dentistry wasn't right for me. It simply wasn't going to be challenging enough, I finally admitted to myself. It wasn't going to satisfy my increasing desire to do something really special with my life, if I possibly could. I didn't yet know what aspect of medicine I wanted to be part of, but now, at least, I knew absolutely that I wanted to be a physician.

I had completed four years of college by that point and had done well, and this time the admissions department at the University of Kansas School of Medicine welcomed me. I was delighted. The medical school was still in Lawrence in those days, but Shaaron was working in Kansas City and we were at home there, so during my first year I lived in a dorm in Lawrence and drove the forty miles home on weekends. It wasn't an ideal situation, but it was acceptable, and right from the outset I knew I'd made the best decision.

Few people who have attended medical school remember it as anything other than a blur—a time during which you're alternately fascinated and overwhelmed, excited and humbled, inspired and exhausted—and for me it was all those things. It was a time, too, when my future in medicine began to take clear shape, yet also a time when I remained uncertain about the physician I wanted to be. I hadn't received lots of hands-on experience at the University of Kansas medical school, and for that reason, as I was about to graduate, I looked for an excellent rotating internship in which I'd really dive into obstetrics, pediatrics, internal medicine, surgery, and a host of specialties. I felt certain that I'd discover an area of medicine that seemed exactly right for me at a big public hospital that was part of a university system, and when I was accepted into a residency at Dallas's Parkland Memorial Hospital, which was affiliated with the University of Texas's Southwestern Medical School, I was thrilled.

Moving to Texas meant moving away from my extended family, of course, but I presumed I'd return to Kansas at some point, and by this time I was ready for the life and career adventure I'd never had before.

On July 1, 1962, I began my first rotation—it was urology, I remember, and almost immediately I was invited into the operating room by the senior resident, Terry Allen, to observe surgery, then to do some surgery myself. I'd developed some surgical skills as part of my research in medical school, but this was the real thing, and I was excited and I did a good job. Yet I was also attracted to obstetrics and gynecology—and neurosurgery had caught my attention as well. It was becoming clear that I liked the kinds of physical procedures that urology, obstetrics, and surgery offered in common: I liked working with my hands, in other words. And when I began to work with a talented young group of general surgery residents at Parkland, I really got turned on. Before the year was out, I knew I wanted to be a

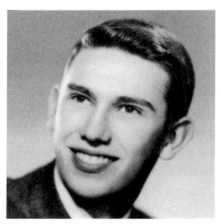

Dr. Salyer as a young medical school graduate

surgeon. I applied for a surgery residency at Parkland—the few available positions were highly competitive, but I was offered one—so the year I'd initially planned to spend in Dallas ultimately became five, and those years changed my life in ways I couldn't have imagined at the time.

I've always been very motivated by colleagues who strive for excellence and who bring passion to their work and their mentoring. Those were the kinds of surgeons under whom I trained in Dallas, and with each surgery rotation, I became ever more convinced that I had the aptitude, hand-eye coordination, and temperament that could help me become a good surgeon. And like my mentors, I had the burning desire to succeed that is almost impossible to teach.

By the fall of 1963, I had completed rotations in general surgery and vascular surgery and was rotating in neurosurgery—something I was enjoying very much—when it was announced locally that President John F. Kennedy would visit Dallas and Fort Worth in a few weeks. I wasn't particularly political, but something about the new president's idealism and call to service to all Americans had moved me powerfully at his inauguration. His election seemed to signal a bright new era in the United States, one filled with hope and possibility, and as for many people in their twenties, for me the president was a heroic figure—larger than life, certainly, yet also someone you could look to for example and inspiration. The president had called on each of us to make a difference in our country and the world, and as a young surgeon in training I felt I was doing my part to answer his call.

I remember that despite the president's limited popularity in Texas, almost all of us at Parkland were exhilarated by the prospect of his visit, and in the cafeteria after early rounds on Friday, November 22, several of us spoke about how much we wished our schedules and responsibilities would allow us to see the president in person during his short visit. Plans had called for him to travel in a motorcade through downtown, not far from Parkland, and we might have caught a glimpse of him at least, but the demands of our rotations kept us away.

It was early afternoon, and I was in an upstairs ward of the hospital when the shocking news began to spread that the president had been shot and had suffered at least one serious wound to the head. One of my neurosurgery rotation duties was to report to the emergency room to assist in head trauma cases, and without waiting to be called, I raced downstairs.

The president was already in the ER when I arrived, and

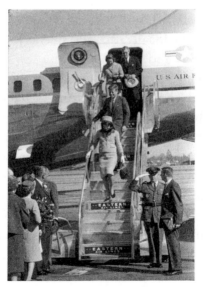

JFK and Jackie arriving at Dallas Love Field

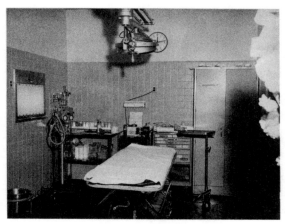

Trauma Room One

Trauma Room One was filling quickly with hospital personnel, secret service officers and police, and even reporters. As I
made my way to the gurney on which President Kennedy lay,
I saw his wife, Jacqueline—wearing the blood-spattered pink
suit that would become so emblematic of that day—standing
in a corner of the room, looking stunned, ashen, and very
much alone.

Already attending to the president was Jim Carrico, a
fellow resident who had been tending to another patient in the
emergency room when Kennedy was wheeled in. Dr. Malcolm
Perry, a vascular surgeon and professor who had become a
friend and mentor, soon joined us as well. We first focused our
attention on getting the president intubated in order to get air
into his lungs. Dr. Carrico wasn't having any success at getting a tube down through the president's nose, so we focused
instead on a small bullet wound in the president's neck
through which he was sucking air. By enlarging the size of the
wound, we ultimately were able to insert a breathing tube into

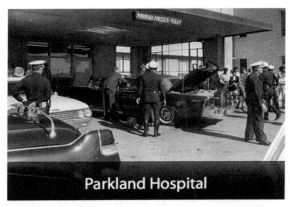

The president's car at Parkland

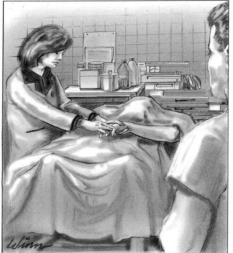

Credit: Bill Winn

An artist's rendering of Dr. Salyer witnessing First Lady Jacqueline Kennedy removing her late husband's wedding ring and placing it on her own finger

the president's lung. Although none of us spoke about it, it was already certain to each of us that anything more we might do to assist the president would be in vain.

The whole right side of Kennedy's cranium had been blown away by a gunshot blast. Much of the right side of his brain had been destroyed as well, and the remainder was exposed by a gaping hole in his skull. The injury was absolutely a fatal one, yet although his brain had been devastated, his heart still beat, and his body continued to reflexively gasp for breath. Our patient was fatally wounded, but he was also the president of the United States, and we were obligated to try every heroic procedure imaginable to save him.

We began to cut away the president's clothes, and I remember my surprise at the size and thickness of the massive brace he wore around his chest and abdomen. I knew the president had suffered a back injury during his service in World War II, but the brace was far more restrictive than anything I might have envisioned. As I cut away the brace, tightly laced like a corset, with heavy shears, it was hard to imagine he could move while wearing it, and it seemed certain that the war injury was far more serious—and painful—than the public knew.

Next, we started an IV line in a vein in his right arm, gave him massive amounts of blood, and continued the oxygen line. Jim Carrico began to vigorously administer external cardiac massage, and when he tired after a long time, I continued it. Aware that the president suffered with Addison's disease—a disorder in which the adrenal glands do not produce sufficient glucocorticoids—we injected the president with steroids, then finally inserted chest tubes, but nothing we did improved his condition in any way. We worked intensely, suggesting to one another anything we might still try, but each of us knew that all hope was lost.

It was impossible to be certain in the horror of the moment

how much time had passed. But after perhaps thirty minutes there was little more we could attempt. Other people in the room sensed the inevitable outcome, and surely the First Lady did as well. I glanced at her in the corner and saw that someone was beside her now, but she continued to stand erect and without assistance, her face expressing both her shock and her profound sorrow.

We had been joined in the ER by Dr. Kemp Clark, the hospital's chief of neurosurgery, and by other senior surgeons and physicians, yet the scene was one of complete helplessness despite the decades of collective experience we brought to our effort. Finally, it was Dr. Clark who reminded us that in addition to attempting to keep the president alive, we shared an obligation to be truthful about his condition. Every monitor attached to his body had flatlined, and Dr. Clark quietly conferred with each of us, then pronounced in a calm but shaken voice, "Gentlemen, President Kennedy has died."

I remember a mass exodus from the room in the moments after the announcement was made. Reporters rushed for telephones, and others simply wandered away in disbelief. But somehow, I couldn't do anything. I had worked with utter focus and without distraction until the pronouncement, but as I heard the words that confirmed the president's death, I could do no more.

As I stood at the table, Mrs. Kennedy approached it, and I remember her looking at me as if to ask if that was okay. I nodded and watched as she moved close to the president's body. She leaned across him to reach for his left hand, removed his wedding ring, and placed it on one of her fingers, and then she simply held her husband's hand in a final good-bye. A priest joined her after a time, gave the president last rites, and then escorted the First Lady out of the room.

I was still standing beside the table, numb and disbelieving, when a few men entered the room with a wooden casket, placed the president's body inside it, then carried him away. I was vividly aware of everything that was going on around me, yet it was as if I were somehow watching from

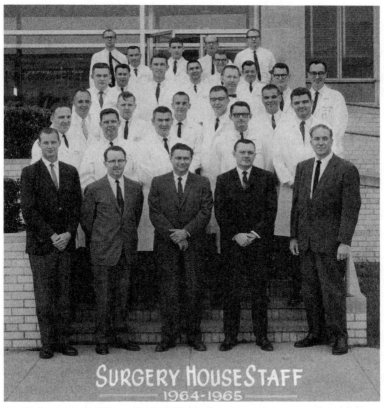

Dr. Salyer (second from the left in the fourth row) as a member of the surgery department at Parkland Hospital, 1964–1965

some distance. But it wasn't long before my numbness was replaced by terrible sadness, by a grief I'd never experienced before. My hero, my champion, a man I had admired and believed in and been hugely inspired by, had died in the hands of my colleagues and me. It was impossible, yet it had happened.

Fifty years later, November 22, 1963, remains a pivotal and powerfully important day in my life, and not simply because fate involved me in one of the most notorious events of the twentieth century. Instead, the president's shooting and my small role in trying to keep him alive offered lessons that were both immediate and have proven to be lifelong.

I was just twenty-seven years old when the president was assassinated, and my career in medicine was still in its infancy. I didn't yet know—really *understand*—how fragile the human body is, in addition to being remarkably resilient. Yet that day, and in the most dramatic way imaginable, I was offered proof that despite medicine's advances and its occasional miracles, death is always only tenuously at bay— for each of us. Like all animals, we live each day of our lives on the precipice of death, whether we're conscious of that reality or not. Yet it's the certainty that death awaits us that gives life its meaning.

And for the first time that day, I realized that while we are well served to keep the certainty of death somewhere in our consciousness, the fear of dying—a fear I continued to carry with me as a constant burden—serves only to limit what we can accomplish while we live. President Kennedy certainly could not have achieved what he did in his forty-six years had his first concern simply been his survival. His military heroism, his work as a public servant, his inspiration of Americans and people around the world to achieve greatness, would have been impossible had he been consumed by the question of when his own death would come. And I realized that if I was to achieve what I hoped to, I'd have to channel the fears that were born in my childhood sickbed into a steely determination to accomplish as much as I could no matter how much time was allowed me.

From that terrible day forward, I realized that John F. Kennedy had led an extraordinary life not because his life was long—it was tragically short—but because of who he had been and what he had accomplished during the time he lived. If I was to have an impact on the world, if *my* life was to matter in

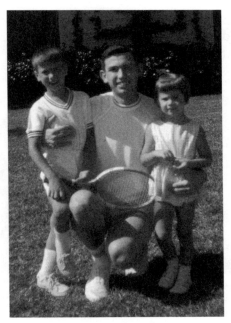

Dr. Salyer with his children, Ken and Leigh

the end, I would have to accept that each succeeding day was all the certainty I'd ever have, and that my job was to make the most of each day, regardless of how many there would be.

I couldn't be certain why, but my long years of fear and illness and uncertainty about my future had long ago kindled in me a desire for my life to have some substance. And then suddenly—and profoundly unexpectedly—the death of my hero before my eyes fanned that quiet desire into a passion. I wanted to live a life of consequence, I somehow *had* to, I now knew. I had to help improve the lives of others, much as he had done, yet in ways that suited my own skills and talents and experience. I didn't yet know the precise path I would take, but I knew it would become my life's mission. I would forge myself into a surgeon who truly made a difference in his patients' lives and perhaps even in the lives of people I'd never meet. My work would matter, I vowed. And so would my life, a life I was eager to live.

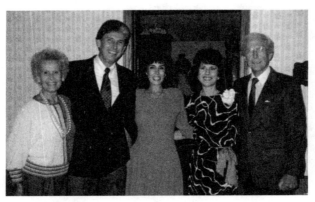

Dr. Salyer with family

Chapter Two

Choosing Plastic Surgery

When Georgette Couvall was born on October 16, 1975, the doctor who delivered her informed her father, "It's a girl, but I've never seen anything like her." It was a horrific thing for a young father to hear, but the obstetrician's lack of tact was nothing compared to the heartbreak both her parents experienced when they were allowed to see her for the first time a few minutes later. Tiny Georgette had a distorted nubbin of a nose and no eye or eye socket on the right side of her face. She had a pronounced overbite and significant difficulty in breathing, and by the time she was a year old, her parents learned that her hearing was compromised as well.

When I first met Georgette, soon after she had turned four, I diagnosed her with a malformation known as frontonasal dysplasia, and I was able to tell her parents that I was sure I could help. Georgette had received some initial surgery in Chicago, where her parents lived, but the results hadn't been what they had hoped—the surgeon was out of his depth and, if anything, had made her circumstances worse. After her mother saw a television segment about the work I was doing in Dallas, her parents became eager for me

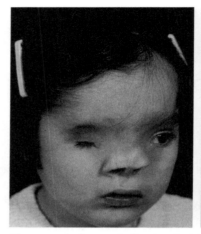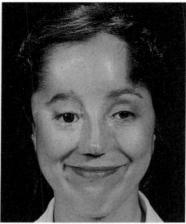

Georgette before and after her facial reconstruction surgery

to meet their daughter and assess her condition and what I might be able to do for her.

A malformation like Georgette's begins sometime during the first few weeks of pregnancy. With a normal fetus, there is a stage in which two bulbs on the side of the head that will become the eyes are very wide-set. Then fusion occurs, drawing the eyes together as the central facial structures develop. So-called neural crest cells proliferate and begin migrating to form the nose, eyes, optic nerves, and supporting structures. But in Georgette's case, this development was mysteriously interrupted and did not continue. Her left eye, vision, and socket developed normally, but the center and right segments of her face were dramatically malformed, including both the soft tissues and the underlying skeletal structure.

I immediately liked Georgette's parents, Jim and Janet Couvall, and shared the delight they took in their daughter, who was old enough by now to know that she wasn't normal, yet who possessed an irrepressible spirit. "Georgette's going to need a number of procedures," I explained to her mom and dad. "None of them will be simple. All of us, and Georgette most of all, will need to remain focused on our long-term goals, but we *can* reach them. Absolutely we can."

I was confident we would succeed because during the decade before I met Georgette, I had become not only a good, well-trained plastic surgeon but also one of the few plastic surgeons in the world who were actively developing an utterly new surgical subspecialty. It would become known as cranio-facial surgery and would allow a small group of us scattered around the world to dramatically improve, and even make normal, the faces of children who, like Georgette, were born with heartbreaking and life-limiting abnormalities.

In the mid-1960s, my internship rotations at Parkland had included a number of different services, and I had developed a passion for general surgery. The Parkland general surgery program operated by the University of Texas Southwestern Medical School was known nationally at that time as a state-of-the-art training enterprise. Its faculty included young, vibrant surgeons like Bob Jones, Bob McClelland, Malcolm Perry, Charlie Baxter, Ron Jones, urologist Paul Peters, oral surgeon Bob Walker, and many others who were passionate about their work and deeply committed to the highest levels of academic medicine.

I was only twenty-seven when I began my general surgery residency, and G. Tom Shires, the chairman of the department, was just eleven years older than me. Easygoing yet determined, he was a fine academic role model for us residents. He became a great friend and a remarkable mentor, one who specialized in the surgical response to traumatic injuries. The program Tom expertly administered demanded a great deal of its residents very quickly. After only a year, during which we rotated among the various general surgery services—vascular, colorectal, trauma, general surgery, and others—under the tutelage of senior residents and the faculty, our second year required us to be in charge of each of the general surgery services on which we rotated. It meant taking real responsibility sooner than some of us wanted it, but it also dramatically strengthened our skills, judgment, and leadership capabilities and provided a remarkable foundation for the rest of our lives as surgeons.

I'll never forget the challenge that commenced on July 1, 1964, when I suddenly was placed in charge of the general surgery service at Parkland. It was among the most dramatic moments of my life, something akin to beginning Navy SEAL training—but already as a commander. And although everything else in my life took a backseat beginning that July—including my family and every other pursuit outside the hospital—it was a once-in-a-lifetime experience that sculpted me and my fellow residents into surgeons with finely honed operating skills, excellent judgment under duress, and the ability to focus on ever-better techniques and procedures that made constant improvement an inherent component of our surgical culture.

As I look back many decades, I think this was perhaps the single most important time in my development as a surgeon. It was mentally and physically demanding in ways only a young and energetic person can withstand, and despite those rigors it cemented in me a profound determination to make surgery my life's work and to grow into a fine surgeon.

In the aftermath of President Kennedy's death, I had a new understanding that life was both fragile and precious, and I became ever more determined to create a professional life that mattered—to me and to those to whom I offered help.

I had been attracted to plastic surgery as a medical student at the University of Kansas when I observed legendary surgeon Dr. David W. Robinson operating on a newborn with a cleft lip and palate, watching as he transformed her in no more than an hour and a half into a normal-looking girl, one whose life would not be compromised by her congenital malformation. I couldn't get that experience out of my head for months afterward, and truthfully, I've carried its memory with me ever since. There was something almost magical in the way the girl's entire future became bright at the hands of Dr. Robinson; it was transformative in a way that seemed almost spiritual then—and it still does.

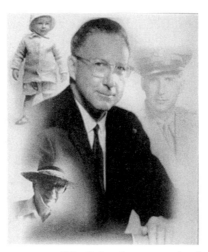

Dr. David Robinson, one of Dr. Salyer's mentors in plastic surgery

I observed that single cleft surgery long before I grew convinced that I wanted to be a plastic surgeon, but I know it influenced me over the succeeding years. At the time, plastic surgery didn't carry with it the prestige that, for example, neurosurgery or cardiac surgery did, but it seemed *important* nonetheless. That child's life had been made whole in a most remarkable way, and I imagined what it would be like to make that endeavor my life's work. And despite my fascination with all kinds of surgery, I kept plastic surgery very much in mind as a career possibility during my years at Parkland—a hospital, as it happened, that didn't have a plastic surgery service—and as a resident at Southwestern Medical School, which didn't offer training in plastic surgery.

The first time I encountered a young patient with a terribly deformed face and skull at Parkland during my general surgery training, I felt totally helpless. I had no skills with which I could offer help, and as far as I knew, nothing anywhere in the world could be done to assist the child. The experience depressed me deeply, and it brought back a flood of memories of how I had felt as a child myself, growing up lonely and rejected. I realized that children and adults with deformed faces must experience such rejection every moment of their lives—a helpless and achingly lonely encapsulation of their entire selves—and it broke my heart to think that nothing could be done for them.

When I announced to my friends, mentors, and fellow residents at Parkland in the spring of 1967 that I would be leaving at the end of the summer to begin a residency in plastic surgery, at first they didn't believe me. Ours was a very macho and competitive world—a surgical culture I was drawn to in many respects—so I wasn't surprised when they reminded me that plastic surgeons occupied a rather humble position in the pantheon of surgical specialties. (Plastic surgeons did menial work; they nipped and tucked; they treated burns and repaired cleft lips and palates, yes, but they didn't operate on brains or hearts) But I wasn't deterred.

I can't really remember how vigorously I defended my decision to become a plastic surgeon, and I'm sure I couldn't have changed their minds in any case. I knew, too, that unlike some surgical specialties, plastic surgery was in its infancy, and that was attractive to me. Unlike some types of surgery, in which there was very clearly only a single way to perform a given procedure, plastic surgery inherently allowed for—even demanded—creativity, and that drew my attention as well. But most of all, for me plastic surgery somehow simply seemed right; it and I were going to be a great fit, I just knew it, and I trusted that instinct.

By now Shaaron and I had two small children—our son, Ken Jr., and our daughter, Leigh, and even in the midst of the myriad challenges and enormous stress of those early years, we had managed to sustain our family life in ways I believed we always would. With my parents' help, we had purchased a three-bedroom home in north Dallas for $16,450, although I didn't get to spend much time there. Often, we held family Sunday dinners in the cafeteria at Parkland because I was on call and was required to be at the hospital. At home, I remember regularly struggling to stay awake in the early evening as I played with the kids before their bedtimes, and night after night I didn't come home at all, catching just an hour or two of sleep at the hospital in a cramped surgeons' lounge before the next day all too soon began.

I did get two weeks of vacation each year during that era, and almost always we used the precious time to drive with a tent trailer mostly to Colorado, but sometimes Wyoming and Montana—places I'd regularly visited with my parents when I was a boy. They were wonderful trips—if always too short. Colorado, in particular, had always been a special place to me, and I wanted to ensure that the kids grew up sharing my love for the Rockies. More than once I imagined living near the mountains one day as a plastic surgeon.

My family had always been important to me, and as I had created a family of my own, I managed to successfully juggle the demands of medical school, internship, and residency with my roles as a husband and a father—at least I thought I did, at least for a while.

I decided to apply for plastic surgery residencies at Duke University, the University of Pennsylvania, the University of Kansas, and at the renowned Johns Hopkins University School of Medicine in Maryland, and I was accepted by all programs. I was funded by a National Institutes of Health traineeship that would provide me with a tax-free stipend wherever I trained. I eagerly accepted the Johns Hopkins position. I was certain it would offer me the best academic opportunity in the country. But before Shaaron and I and the kids could initiate our move to Maryland, my father became seriously ill with encephalitis.

His recovery would be slow, and I wanted to be near him, so I made a decision I've never regretted. I chose family over career—in ways that wouldn't always be the case as my professional life unfolded—and I returned to Kansas City and did my plastic surgery residency under David W. Robinson. Robinson was six feet four inches tall, soft-spoken and dedicated, and I had enormous respect for him. He was a good teacher and a leader in the field of plastic surgery in America, and at that time, Kansas had one of the best plastic surgery programs in the country. Robinson became a true mentor; I identified with him and modeled myself after him in many ways, and under his tutelage I learned state-of-the-art cleft lip and palate surgery, which has fascinated and fulfilled me ever since.

It was great to be back at home in Kansas in the fall of 1967—even though I still had to devote myself to my work for sixteen or so hours every day—and once more I had the opportunity to be mentored by extraordinary surgeons. Dr. Robinson had captivated me with his reconstructive work almost a decade before, and he did once more as I began to be trained by him and by Dr. Frank Masters, whose specialty was what then was more commonly called *cosmetic* surgery. Masters was indeed a master, a surgeon who forcefully made the case that everything I learned about reshaping and contouring "normal" faces and bodies was directly applicable to reconstructive work. He quickly convinced me that the better I became as an aesthetic surgeon, the better surgeon I would be overall. The goal in cleft lip and palate surgery, he pointed out by example, wasn't simply to reconstruct but to reconstruct *aesthetically*, to create a new face for each child that was as attractive as possible.

Yet overall, my residency in plastic surgery at the University of Kansas disappointed me. After my extraordinary experience as a general surgery resident at Parkland, one in which my fellow residents and I were given immediate leadership responsibilities, the more conventional structure of the Kansas program—in which I was a junior resident working under senior residents who had little or no more experience than I did—left me concerned that my plastic surgery training wouldn't ultimately be of the caliber I had hoped.

It was during my residency, too, that I first confronted the fact that a surgeon's life and family life can be difficult to perfectly blend. In the midst of my senior year, during the time I served as chief resident in plastic surgery at KUMC, I suffered a herniated disk in my lower back, an injury caused by regularly lifting burn patients without being careful enough. I developed severe toe and foot pain that I feared might destroy my ability to work on my feet for long hours each day in surgery. I was thirty-two years old, but suddenly I felt like a sick kid again. I was afraid, angry, impatient, and depressed, and I dealt with my fears in ways that were too often inappropriate. My relationship with Shaaron was tested during that time, and although our marriage survived, it became impossible for me to ignore the fact that my career goals and my attraction to the ideals of family life might clash repeatedly in the coming years.

Eventually, I had surgery and the disk was successfully repaired, and I was grateful that I was going to be able to work as a surgeon after all. My outlook on life dramatically improved, and I was even able to secure a prestigious traveling fellowship that would allow me to visit an American surgical center of my choice and spend a month observing distinguished surgeons like Bob Chase and Don Laub at Stanford, Ralph Millard in Miami, Bob McCormack at the University of Rochester in New York, and Gustave Aufricht and John Converse at the New York University Medical Center in Manhattan.

Dr. John Converse was internationally renowned in reconstructive plastic surgery. He had edited a seven-volume plastic surgery text that I had studied; he was well known as a pioneer of surgical techniques—some of which still bear his name—and there was no one I knew from whom I was more eager to learn. My time with him in New York literally changed my life.

I was already a plastic surgeon; I'd already set the course of my career in that regard, but it wasn't until I met and observed Dr. Converse in the heady environment of the Institute of Reconstructive Plastic Surgery at NYU's Langone Medical Center that I realized I wanted to be an explorer as well. I didn't simply want to perform long-established procedures throughout my career; I wanted, like Dr. Converse, to be an innovator, to study, experiment, test, and not only

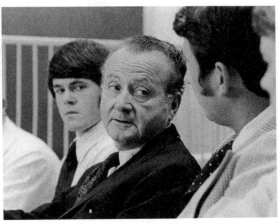

Dr. Salyer was influenced by Dr. John Converse while in New York in 1969

assist specific patients but also help move plastic surgery forward into the future. I learned during my brief time in New York that I had been wrong when I despaired that nothing could be done to help children with tragic facial deformities or people who had suffered head and facial injuries. At NYU, Dr. Converse was pioneering new techniques that were *working*, and I wanted to follow in his footsteps. I returned to Kansas with a vision of the shape my life's work would take, thrilled by the possibilities and secure in the knowledge that, like John Converse, I could help give disfigured children the gift of a normal face.

Sometimes life really does have its significant moments. On June 30, 1969, I completed my plastic surgery residency at the University of Kansas, and the following day I became the first professor and chairman of the new division of plastic surgery in the department of surgery at the University of Texas's Southwestern Medical School.

As the Vietnam War escalated during my years of surgical training, I'd received a Berry Plan draft deferment that allowed me to complete my training and then enter the air force as a commissioned lieutenant, followed by two years of service as an air force surgeon. But because of my herniated disk, I failed my induction physical in the spring of 1969. The air force no longer wanted me, but it turned out that my former mentor Tom Shires, the head of the surgery department at UT's Southwestern Medical School, did.

Southwestern's surgery department had for a long time lacked a plastic surgery division—a significant hole in an otherwise outstanding program—and I was honored and very pleased when Tom contacted me to inquire whether I'd be interested in returning to Texas, this time not as an intern or a resident but as a professor, working with the same team of surgeons and medical professionals who had inspired, supported, and guided me a few years before. I eagerly said yes to the offer; Shaaron and I and the kids headed south to Dallas again—a city we already knew we liked and where we had established enduring friendships. I was about to turn thirty-three, and for the first time in my life, I would no longer be a student or in an advanced level of training. I would hold a salaried academic position; I'd have the opportunity to create a plastic surgery division from the ground up, and I knew I'd have the support of my superiors to make it excellent in every way. Perhaps most importantly, I would have the opportunity to play an important role in advancing the development of plastic surgery of the head and face, a role that would potentially extend my reach far beyond Dallas. I was thrilled.

So on the sultry first day of July 1969, I arrived at Parkland hospital with the sense that I was about to begin a career track on which I might well remain for the rest of my life. It was a humble beginning—my domain consisted of a bare-bones research lab, a tiny office, and a single secretarial assistant. Yet before two years had passed, we had made great strides, working closely with Charlie Baxter at Parkland's already renowned burn center, providing the opportunity to expand the plastic surgery service, and developing Texas's first children's pediatric plastic surgery department at Dallas's Children's Medical Center, as well as founding, in conjunction with Drs. Mutaz Habal and Bob Parsons, a section of pediatric plastic surgery at the American Academy of Pediatrics.

In addition to performing hundreds of surgical procedures

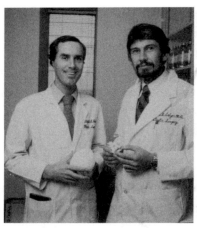

In the research laboratory with Ralph Holmes

each year, now I was also a professor and program administrator. If my schedule had been intensely busy in the years before, now it was even more demanding. Research, publication, hospital committees, national conferences, and extensive travel had become part of my regular responsibilities as well. I was swamped with work, but it was work I loved, and it was hard to imagine a richer life or one more suited to my talents and passions.

When I returned to New York in 1971 to observe NYU's Dr. John Converse in surgery again, I was introduced to his friend and colleague Dr. Paul Tessier, a French reconstructive surgeon who already was something of a legend among plastic surgeons around the world. At Dr. Converse's invitation, Dr. Tessier had traveled to New York from Paris to perform an operation on a young patient with a complex and highly disfiguring congenital disorder called Crouzon's syndrome. Crouzon's occurs when an infant's skull and facial bones begin to fuse in utero and normal bone development cannot occur, resulting in radically abnormal patterns of skull and facial growth. Crouzon's sufferers often have short, broad heads that are very narrow from front to back, and widely set and bulging eyes.

The surgery lasted thirteen hours. Dr. Tessier and his team worked tirelessly—and brilliantly, it seemed to me— reshaping the child's skull with remodeling and forehead advancement, rebuilding her eye sockets and repositioning her eyes, and simultaneously moving her upper face and maxilla, the upper jaw, forward in a procedure that became known as a Le Fort III. I knew as I watched Dr. Tessier operate that his extraordinary skills held the answer for all the children I had seen at Children's Medical Center in Dallas whom I'd been unable to help. It was an electrifying moment, one in which I saw irrefutable evidence that the skeletal structure and soft tissues of the head and face could be dramatically transformed with techniques and instruments that existed *now*. I was glimpsing the future, but quite wonderfully, it was a future that was unfolding in the present moment, and it solidified my belief that I had found my surgical niche.

Nineteen years older than me, Paul Tessier had been born in a town on the French Atlantic coast into a family of wine merchants and had entered medical school in 1936, the year I was born. He became a prisoner of war in 1940, during the German occupation of France, and while incarcerated became critically ill with a typhoid infection of the heart. He was released from prison and recovered, but two years later he escaped death a second time when he opted to join medical students he was mentoring for a picnic a half hour before an American bombing raid destroyed the hospital where he was working in the city of Nantes.

As I had, Tessier had become interested in facial deformity and the possibilities for its surgical correction when he was introduced to cleft lip and palate surgery. He moved to Paris at the end of the war and joined the pediatric service at Hôpital Foch, where he began to specialize in plastic surgery of the head and face—a specialization that later would spur him to undertake his groundbreaking work.

He began traveling to England frequently, where surgeons Sir Harold Gillies and Sir Archibald McIndoe were making great advances in plastic surgery in response to the injuries suffered by English soldiers during the war. By the mid-1950s, Tessier had become the head of his department in Paris, and in 1957 he met a child with Crouzon's syndrome whose upper jaw and eye sockets were so poorly developed that his bulging eyes threatened to cause blindness and his breathing was dangerously obstructed. At the time, neither Gillies, McIndoe, nor anyone else in the world was capable of helping him, but Tessier was determined to find a way. Gillies had performed the first Le Fort III facial advancement in 1953 but came away convinced that the surgery should never be performed again. Tessier, on the other hand, was confident he could perform the surgery, and the French child gave him an opportunity to prove it.

Believing there had to be a method by which the lower eye sockets and jaw could be surgically liberated from the skull, then moved into more normal positions, Tessier initially experimented with dry skulls but was denied access to work with cadavers by the Paris medical establishment, which considered his goal little more than folly. Tessier was not easily discouraged, and he leaped that hurdle by regularly traveling by train to Nantes in the evening, where he would work late into the night with cadavers, then return to Paris in the early hours of the following morning for the next day's work. He ultimately became confident enough that he performed an initial surgery on the child, advancing the face of the Crouzon's patient by twenty-five millimeters and stabilizing it with grafts from the patient's own rib bone.

It was an immense achievement, and news of it spread rapidly around the world. Yet more fame soon would follow. Within three years, Tessier and French neurosurgeon Gérard Guiot jointly devised a technique for surgically separating the eye sockets from the frontal bone of the skull, an astonishing procedure that made it possible to reposition eyeballs that were abnormally wide-set (a condition known as hypertelorism), bringing them closer together by cutting and translocating the orbits containing the eyes.

These were revolutionary surgeries, and the fact that Tessier proved they were possible meant that many kinds of facial anomalies might soon be successfully treated, transforming the treatment of craniofacial birth defects, cancers of the face and skull, and severe facial asymmetries. By 1967, when he hosted an international symposium devoted to explication and demonstration of the new procedures, interest in Tessier's work among plastic surgeons around the world was enormous. Paris emerged as the locus of the new specialty called craniofacial surgery, and Paul Tessier was, without doubt, its progenitor.

From my own perspective, something that was particularly exciting about Tessier's advances was their interlinking of plastic surgeries, maxillofacial surgeries, ophthalmic surgeries, and neurosurgeries. Each specialty had increasingly important things to offer the other—and I was certain all of them would benefit far into the future. Tessier, too, was a strong advocate for the importance of aesthetics as a fundamental goal in each patient's treatment, and that was a perspective I readily shared. He was never content for a patient simply to look somewhat better than he or she did before surgery. "If it is not normal it is not enough," he unstintingly proclaimed.

I had been elated to watch Dr. Tessier work, and that experience directly led to my decision in 1971 to perform my first craniofacial surgery on a young girl with Treacher Collins syndrome—a genetic disorder commonly characterized by downward-slanting eyes; small, underdeveloped jawbones and cheekbones; small or absent ears; attendant hearing loss; and drooping lower eyelids. I opened the girl's scalp above her hairline, then peeled down her face; I then used pieces of her ribs, which I carved and contoured, to reconstruct her face. The results were good; she did well postoperatively, and I was delighted to see her again many years later and observe how close to Tessier's standard of normalcy I had come with my first major case.

At the time, I was one of only a handful of surgeons around the world who was responding to Tessier's challenge to innovate with pioneering work of our own. You can imagine how excited I was in May 1972 to be invited to Paris for a week during which I would join surgeons like me from several countries in observing Tessier and his team and gleaning as much knowledge as I could to help me back at home.

Besides observing Dr. Tessier in the operating room for a week, I was able to enjoy his company at meetings and dinners. For a boy from Kansas making his first visit to Europe, the trip was eye-opening in every way. Tessier was a great conversationalist, sportsman, wine connoisseur, and gourmand, and I couldn't help being a little in awe of his intellect, energy, and passion for his work. The surgeons he had invited were a fascinating group as well. Daniel Marchac, based in Paris, was observing Tessier as his young protégé and was already a remarkable surgeon himself; Jack Mustardé, a Scot living and working in Glasgow, had built an international reputation as an ophthalmic plastic surgeon; Linton Whitaker and Ian Munro were innovative young plastic surgeons based in Philadelphia and Toronto, respectively; and Fernando Ortiz Monasterio was an urbane, witty, and altogether captivating surgeon focusing on craniofacial surgery in Mexico City, where he had already established an internationally well-respected plastic surgery clinic and training center.

Fernando was thirteen years older than me—and a dozen times worldlier—and our friendship was instantaneous. He took me under his wing, introduced me to the glories of Paris and the pleasures of French wine and escargots, and I loved his boundless enthusiasm for the future of our field. He and Tessier had become good friends some years before—Fernando's French was as good as his English—and it wasn't uncommon for him to fly all night from Mexico City, spend a full day operating with Tessier, have a long and convivial dinner with him, then fly home to Mexico City on a second red-eye flight so he could punctually return to his own work. Fernando specialized in reconstructive and aesthetic surgery, and like Tessier, he was an innovator and an aesthetician as well as an excellent technical surgeon. By the early 1990s, he would become the most famous plastic surgeon in the world.

I went home to Dallas after a life-changing experience in Paris and began to plan, work with cadavers, and slowly but surely create new surgical techniques that could help the children I had had to turn away before, children like Charlotte Allison, who had Robinow syndrome, which resulted in her having a small, underdeveloped face, a dramatic frontal protrusion of the forehead, overly wide-set eyes, and a stubby, upturned nose.

Soon after returning from Paris, I began to focus on what would be a tremendously complex surgery for Charlotte—planning in detail its execution, reading about and discussing related cases with colleagues far and wide, and experimenting with cadavers. By September, I believed I was ready to try to change the life of this girl, who lived in terrible seclusion, and together with Ron Atkins, my resident in plastic surgery; Dr. Maurice Saunders, the sole pediatric neurosurgeon in Dallas at the time; and Rosalyn Patterson—my extraordinary scrub nurse, a petite South Texas dynamo who would work intrepidly at my side for the subsequent twenty-five years—I performed the first intracranial hypertelorism correction in the southwestern United States.

In those days, we had no CT scans, no MRIs, and no three-dimensional modeling, and it was a tremendous challenge to perform the thirteen-hour procedure, one that lasted well into the night. But the operation was both a great success and a vital moment in my career, one that satisfied me that I had the commitment, talent, and skills to work at the highest levels and embark on advanced and highly complex surgery that many of my peers would remain reluctant to undertake for some time. I became utterly focused on developing these techniques on my own, driven by my longstanding desire for perfection, on the one hand, and a personal emotional need to help children who were rejected by society and lived in heartbreaking seclusion on the other. (And what a gratifying day it was many years later to attend the wedding of lovely Charlotte Allison, whose life now was unfolding in wonderful ways.)

A young patient named Lynn Beaver had been a similar recluse, someone who even some members of her extended family did not know existed. Lynn had the love and support of her parents, but they were convinced that any sort of normal life was impossible for her, so they protectively kept her almost entirely at home in ways that made me ache for her. A Crouzon's patient, Lynn had dangerously bulging eyes, a misshapen skull, a retruded upper jaw, and a protruding lower jaw. Surgery would be essential if her eyesight was to be saved, and with a number of surgeries over time, I felt confident I could give Lynn a normal face.

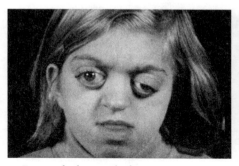 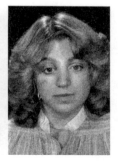

Lynn Beaver before and after surgery

But Lynn's case was complex; I needed every bit of assistance and support I could muster, and fortunately for both of us, in 1974 Dr. Tessier accepted my invitation to come to Dallas to attend an international symposium I was hosting on plastic surgery of the orbital region surrounding the eye. No one in the world had more experience with Crouzon's surgeries than Paul Tessier, and during his time in Dallas, Dr. Tessier joined me in operating on six of my patients— Lynn included. Not only did her initial surgery go as well as I'd hoped it would, but my Dallas team and I also learned an enormous amount that week from the now-heralded father of the subspecialty that had become our focal work as well. The experience was a bit like taking piano lessons from Beethoven, and everyone in Dallas with whom I regularly worked—from neurosurgeons to surgery techs—was able to see for themselves that the stories they long had heard from me about Tessier's technical and creative brilliance were true.

I was developing something of a reputation of my own by the mid-1970s, and Dallas was joining Paris and a few other

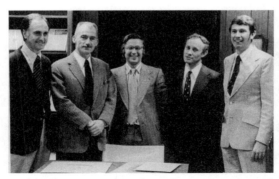

Dr. Salyer with colleague-surgeons in Dallas, 1974 (Drs. Whitaker, Tessier, Ian Jackson, Munro, and Salyer)

cities as focal locations for cutting-edge reconstructive surgery. I had established myself as a very capable cleft lip and palate surgeon, and now I was also successfully reshaping the heads and faces of children with Crouzon's and other genetic disorders, successfully experimenting in the laboratory as well as the operating room with bone grafts, bone healing and replacement, and synthetic bone substitutes— all of which had immediate and future importance in reconstruction.

For almost a decade, I'd also had an ongoing interest in microsurgery—surgery performed with the aid of microscopes to allow anastomosis (reconnection) of blood vessels and nerves only a few millimeters in diameter, making it increasingly possible to transfer tissue from one part of a patient's body to another. In the early 1970s, microsurgery had only been accomplished in the laboratory and, like craniofacial surgery, was in its relative infancy. Hand surgeons at the University of Louisville performed the first revascularization of a partially amputated finger in 1963—the first time minute blood vessels had been reconnected successfully enough for blood to flow through them again. And in 1964, well-known plastic surgeon Dr. Harry J. Buncke reported the experimental replantation of a rabbit's ear after it had been severed, paving the way for similar reconstructive work with humans soon thereafter. If I hadn't initially become fascinated by the possibilities of craniofacial surgery at NYU in 1969, I might well have become a microsurgeon myself, but by the 1970s, the instruments and techniques for a number of surgical subspecialties had begun to merge, and many reconstructive plastic surgeons like me were developing expertise not only with soft tissue but also with bone and blood vessels, and working inside the skull alongside neurosurgeons.

It was a wonderfully expansive time; new procedures were being developed almost every month, it sometimes seemed, and their effects on patients' lives were enormous. It was a heady time to be a surgeon, and I focused intensely on my work—too often to the exclusion of everything else in my life—building a name for myself in Texas, then later throughout the United States and around the world.

During the 1974 Dallas symposium that Tessier attended, I suggested to several of the young surgeons whom I had met in Paris two years before that we form an international craniofacial club, one that would allow us to rendezvous at least once a year, present to each other our most challenging cases and our newest techniques and advances, and solicit help with the problems we couldn't yet solve, as well as enjoy some recreational time together. Ian Jackson from Scotland, working at the famous Cannesburn Plastic Surgery Hospital at the time; Ian Munro; and Linton Whitaker immediately liked the idea. Daniel Marchac in Paris soon joined us, as did Fernando Ortiz Monasterio, and the frequent rendezvous proved to be a real boom to each of us. In that pre-Internet and pre-email era, our ability to communicate regularly at our meetings about the work we were doing helped me immensely, and I know it did the others as well. It wasn't the same as if we had been on staff at the same hospital, of course, but it fostered the support, camaraderie, and friendly competition that is a vital part of how medical and surgical advancements are made.

For several decades to come, and despite our separate and chaotically busy schedules, we succeeded in meeting once a

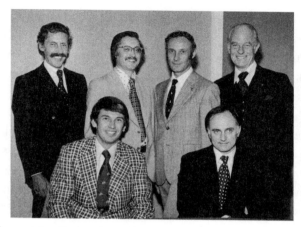

Dr. Salyer with colleague-surgeons

year or more in various places around the world, presenting our cases, discussing complications, and doing our best to follow admirably in the footsteps of our mentor, Dr. Tessier. Much of what we presented to one another we also published for wide dissemination in the journal *Plastic and Reconstructive Surgery* and other important publications. The four of us who were native English speakers—Ian Jackson, Ian Munro, Linton Whitaker, and I—wrote and edited the first *Atlas of Craniomaxillofacial Surgery* ever published, which became the de facto bible of the nascent subspecialty, and it was a sign of our collective success that we were increasingly invited to present at prestigious international meetings of organizations whose scope was broader than our own, such as the Plastic Surgery Research Council, the Clemson Bioengineering Society, and the American College of Surgeons.

Each of the six of us had his own areas of particular expertise; we shared our knowledge and frustrations, successes and failures in equal measure, and I'm proud when I think of the numbers of children whose lives were transformed on our operating tables and at the hands of the hundreds of other surgeons of subsequent generations each of us trained over the years.

Georgette Couvall was one of those children who might have lived a very different life if she had been born just a few years earlier. If Paul Tessier hadn't initiated a new surgery that was revolutionary, and if surgeons like my five far-flung colleagues and I hadn't been shown the way by him, or hadn't been brave enough to make daring advances of our own, Georgette might have grown up as an outcast and with very little hope for a full life. That wasn't the case, of course, and Georgette and I became a team. Together we accomplished something of which we both remain very proud.

Besides the challenges of her appearance, Georgette's condition posed serious health issues as well. She not only had no structural nose on her right side, but she also suffered from choanal nasal passage atresia—the back of her nasal passage was closed, blocked by abnormal bony and soft tissue that had formed during her fetal development. A Chicago surgeon had attempted to correct the problem and had been partially successful. But no effort had been made yet to build a nose, and that was in our favor—the several doctors who had treated her just didn't have the skills for such intricate and complex work. Her parents were discouraged, but they certainly hadn't given up hope, and Georgette was fortunate that they were determined to find the best care for their daughter they could.

At our first meeting, Georgette's mother, Janet, told me

they were concerned about finding the right physician to place in charge of her daughter's future treatment. Janet's confidence had been shaken by her experiences in Chicago, and she and her husband, Jim, planned to meet with me and two other plastic surgeons—both of whom I knew and highly respected. Decisions about a child's care, particularly when surgery is involved, are very difficult for families like Georgette's, and it's important that they feel very comfortable with their choices.

After consultations with a number of other doctors, Georgette's family ultimately decided to return to see me, and I think perhaps it was somehow meant to be that I would take charge of her care. Yet I couldn't have known as we set out that I would ultimately perform *thirteen* operations on that brave young woman. From the outset, I knew that her case was very difficult, and to be honest, as I began I didn't know precisely how I was going to achieve an acceptable reconstruction of her face.

Georgette was an all-too-perfect example of the multitude of problems a reconstructive plastic surgeon commonly faces in his or her effort to reconstruct a major deformity, whether congenital, acquired, traumatic, or caused by a tumor. With Georgette, I knew I would have to consider at length each step of her reconstruction; there was no existing road map, nor any recognized "plan" that would neatly suit her situation. At that period in my career, in each case I took on, I would first address the problem, then study, read, and plan in an attempt to determine the best method, technique, steps, and sequencing that I believed would lead to the optimal result. It was an era when I was mentally developing techniques at the same time my hands were executing them, and it was a simple matter of gaining experience and recognizing that very seldom was there a single answer or a single approach to any problem.

In Georgette's case, I determined that she was a craniofacial patient who presented hard-tissue and soft-tissue deformities that had to be repaired step by meticulous step, borrowing bone and tissue from other parts of her body as needed, in the attempt to reconstruct a four-year-old face into contours that I was confident would be aesthetically pleasing once she was grown.

One of the most difficult problems for any plastic surgeon is reconstructing a growing face. If one were to create—or could create—the perfect nose on a four-year-old, it would be totally inadequate when that child became an adult. The great challenge is for a surgeon to use his or her acquired science, art, and fund of experience to achieve not simply a correction but a functioning, acceptable, and even beautiful face. My goal with Georgette was to allow the beauty already within her to emerge, as well as to protect her from society's harsh judgment of the mask of deformity that currently shrouded her.

This was a very big challenge for my expertise—or anyone's. Georgette had many missing parts, a very misshapen face, totally inadequate tissue with which to build her nose, tiny eyelids, a deformed bony orbit without an eye, and abnormal occlusion of her jaws and teeth; nor did she have adequate facial bone structure to form the necessary framework on which to construct a normal face. The tasks would be overwhelming except for the possibility of addressing them one at a time. I decided for the time being to ignore Georgette's abnormal skeletal framework and first concentrate on reconstruction of the eyelids, then build from there.

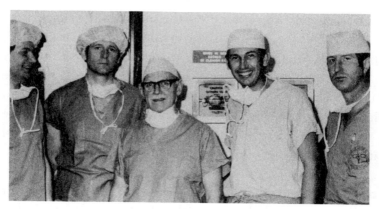

Dr. Salyer, Dr. Mustardé, and residents

At four years old, she was older than I would have liked as I began to detail her treatment. As a general rule, the younger a child with a major craniofacial deformity is when he or she undergoes surgery, the better the long-term outcome. In consultation with my colleague and friend in Scotland, Dr. Jack Mustardé—who had begun his career as an ophthalmologist and who specialized in reconstruction of the areas surrounding the eyes—during the first operation, I focused on her missing right eyelids. She did have vestigial lids, and this was very much in our favor, because an eyelid contains the eyelashes, which are almost impossible to duplicate, and both lids and lashes perform vital functions in protecting the eye and keeping it moist, in addition to being very important aesthetically.

Reshaping and repairing this type of deformity is extremely complicated, in largest part because it involves disparate types of tissue. The skin at the margin of the eyelid is made up of squamous cells, but on the inside of the lid the skin is very tightly attached to the conjunctiva—the mucous membrane that covers the front of the eye and lines the inside of the eyelids. There is also a cartilaginous structure in the eyelid that supports the eye itself, which is very difficult to duplicate. In this case, I was attempting to create a more normal upper eyelid by moving a flap of the vestigial lower eyelid about five millimeters up and suturing it to the upper eyelid, temporarily supplying blood to the area until it became vascularized.

It was the first of a whole series of intricate operations: creating the upper eyelid from the lower, creating the lower eyelid from skin taken from the cheek by rotating it into position, creating the lining of the lid by extending tissue that was there, and using a separate graft of mucosa to create the inside lining of the lower eyelid. Later I added cartilage from Georgette's nose to create the support for her newly reconstructed lower eyelid.

Next came medial and lateral canthopexies—tendon-tightening procedures to reinforce the position of the lower eyelid. This helped to align Georgette's new upper and lower right eyelids with her left eye so that she would have two normal-looking eyes once a prosthetic eye was added.

In addition to constructing a socket and lids for the right eye prosthesis, I made a small incision in the corner of Georgette's normal left eye, removing a small amount of bone and moving both the left and right medial canthi in an effort to ensure that they were on an identical horizontal level. And in the midst of all of these small steps focused on her eyelids, I was also taking preliminary steps to create a nose.

Although she would never be able to see from it, of course, it was exciting to approach the point when we would give

Georgette her new right eye. As initial steps toward that end, in a series of small surgeries I had taken skin and cartilage from her ear and inner thigh to create the structure of the lower eyelid that would support the weight and shape of the prosthetic eye. From the time of the earliest forms of plastic surgery practiced by Italian surgeon Gasparo Tagliacozzi in the sixteenth century, plastic surgeons have always had to borrow tissue and bone from their patients to create and nurture the successful implantation of new structures. It's one of the thousand miracles of human growth and development that, given sufficient blood supply, skin and bone grow remarkably well when transplanted elsewhere in one's body, and with Georgette it was certain from the outset of her treatment that *her* gifts would be as important as mine or anyone else's in achieving the transformation we sought.

I coordinated my work with an ocularist who fashioned a prosthetic eye specifically for Georgette, one that matched her left eye as closely as possible. As was the case with virtually every other element of Georgette's multiyear treatment, successfully implanting the new eye was a challenge. Her lids had to be sewn closed and the area left alone for a number of months to allow the graft to grow and maintain expansion, and there was always the danger that the newly constructed socket would shrink during that period. And there was no guarantee that every element would fit properly after the initial procedure; it isn't uncommon to have to repeat it to achieve an optimal result. The eye, the lids, and their movements are fantastically complex, and we all were delighted when, at the end of a four-month wait, Georgette's new eye fit perfectly and looked great.

I remember how excited Georgette was on the day she

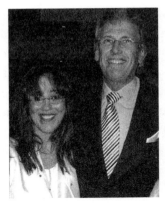

Georgette with Dr. Salyer years after her surgeries

stood in front of a mirror, seeing for the first time a face with *two* bright eyes as she radiantly smiled at the face she observed. It was a wonderful moment. "I look like a *real* girl," she said with great delight.

She was in kindergarten by then, and she had begun to share with her parents and me the kinds of taunts she received from other kids—teasing that tore at her parents' hearts as well as mine. Kids can be cruel, of course, and we remained a long way from completing the process of giving Georgette the normal—and beautiful—face that this delightful little girl deserved, but we had made great progress, and her smile was proof of it.

Georgette would have to endure much more—in the hospital and out in the world as well—but she was both patient and brave, and I remember very clearly that I took real strength from *her* during those days because, like her, I was facing trials that, at times, I wasn't sure I could bear.

I had succeeded by the end of the 1980s in becoming one

of the top half dozen craniofacial surgeons in the world, and it was an accomplishment of which I was rightfully proud. I had devoted myself virtually obsessively to achieving excellence in my craft; I had pushed myself relentlessly and had proved my worth to myself—and I had always been my most demanding critic. I'd become capable of offering patients like Georgette new lives, but I had paid a demanding price in my own.

My marriage—once the most secure and important element in my life—had fallen apart, and neither Shaaron nor I could find a way to repair it. I now had to confront the fact that divorce had become a certainty.

I had been instrumental in developing a national reputation for the division of plastic surgery at Southwestern Medical School. I'd established the first formal residency training program in plastic surgery in the Dallas–Fort Worth area and had also created a strong pediatric plastic surgery service at Children's Medical Center of Dallas, where I was establishing the first craniofacial center in the Southwest. We were doing pioneering work and expanding constantly, but then—quite suddenly and terribly—all of that appeared to be gone as well.

It was unimaginable, but just as my career was reaching heights I might never have envisioned, it appeared that it was being taken from me. My marriage was over; and now, it seemed, my career was, too, and I wasn't sure how I could go on.

Chapter Three

Building a Dream

My childhood years had been difficult, but in the two decades since I had gone to college and set my sights on a career in medicine, I had seemed singularly blessed. I'd married a wonderful woman and was raising two children whom I adored. I'd received the best medical and surgical training anyone could hope for, and, by the time I reached forty, I had become not only a full professor of surgery and the chairman of the division of plastic surgery at the University of Texas Southwestern Medical School, but I was also one of just a handful of surgeons around the world who were building international reputations in the new field of craniofacial surgery. My good fortune was beyond any dream I could have mustered during the years I spent sick and in solitude as a child, greater than any I could have imagined as I determined, after President Kennedy's assassination, to find a path toward a life of real consequence.

But as I turned forty-two, that good fortune utterly left my life. My long marriage fell to pieces and ended miserably. My family was torn apart and I was deeply saddened, and then—unimaginably—I was fired from the position I had hoped I would hold throughout my entire career. Quite suddenly, *everything* that had given my life personal and professional stability was gone. All my accomplishments seemed to count for very little, and I struggled to believe there was a way I could possibly put my life back together.

In retrospect, the collapse of my marriage was not unlike the demise of many marriages in which one or both partners are consumed by intensely demanding and stressful professional lives. Physicians and surgeons have far from the best marriage survival statistics in the world, and the reasons are obvious, perhaps, but in my case that didn't make them any less painful. The loss of my job, on the other hand, was something that rarely happens to someone in a position like mine, and when it does, its consequences are often devastating for years to come. Throughout my medical career till this point, I had been something of a wunderkind, achieving great success while I was still quite young. But now I was alone, out of work, depressed, and defeated, and I had to face the real possibility that my career as a craniofacial surgeon was over.

During the years I had administered the division of plastic surgery at Southwestern and developed it into a program of national prominence, I had often struggled with my administrative superiors to secure what I believed was a level of funding necessary to achieve true excellence. We were accomplishing great things with very limited resources, and my constant requests for increased program funds, salaries, and professional travel stipends were virtually never met with approval.

I had never been someone who could readily accept the limitations of rules and regulations, always aggressively desiring to expand the envelope of what we could accomplish in plastic surgery and pushing back against ways of operating that seemed unnecessarily restrictive and counterproductive to the medical school's stated goals, my own career, and opportunities to do something big and bold.

The plastic surgery division I was in charge of was by now generating nearly three million dollars in revenue annually, which had to be turned over to the chancellor of the university to be used as he saw fit. At many other schools around the country, program administrators like me were able to control a significant percentage of the funds they generated to use for development and expansion of their own divisions. I thought that made great sense, but my boss, Charles Sprague, the chancellor of the university's Health Science Center, strongly disagreed. He and I struggled continuously to find common ground, but I was young and headstrong and more than a little taken with my early success. He, on the other hand, believed foremost—it seemed to me—in the sanctity of doing things by the book. He was commanding and authoritarian and he didn't want a freethinker administering the plastic surgery division that was a key component of his domain, didn't want a cowboy in charge whom he couldn't control, and he ultimately had to have my head. It was entirely in his power to fire me, which he suddenly and very dramatically did, and I had no way to appeal his decision or persuade him to change it.

I was living in a dingy one-bedroom apartment at the time, missing the family life Shaaron and I and the kids had created over the previous twenty years. And now, with this shocking defeat—one I had personally set in motion with my determination to bend rules and do things *my* way—I was devastated. I fell into a deep depression, convinced that my career in academic plastic surgery was finished. Academia, craniofacial surgery, and my two children were my greatest loves, and although the kids were not lost to me, nowadays I saw them far less than I wanted. I believed I had terribly let them down, as I had my colleagues in the plastic surgery division who had worked so passionately with me to create something special, and I'd failed my patients as well.

As far as I now could envision, my future would necessarily be limited to private practice and a focus on cosmetic surgery if I was to make ends meet financially, send my kids to college, pay alimony, and meet my other expenses in the years ahead. I felt certain that craniofacial and academic plastic surgery were simply gone from my life. My professional life no longer would include publication in academic journals, the training and mentoring of young surgeons, or stimulating relationships with other craniofacial surgeons around the world as we jointly strove to expand the boundaries of our still-new subspecialty. Nothing mattered more to me than those things, but because of decisions I alone had made, they were gone forever. I had fulfilled my dreams, and now I had destroyed them.

It's hard to know how one goes about recovering from a massive defeat, harder still for someone like me to offer advice on how to do it. But I recognize as I look back on that time—which without question was the most difficult time of my life—that at some point I simply was finished with the self-loathing that seemed to engulf me for too long, finished also with depression and the need to relive the past and the role I had played in my own defeat.

A day simply arrived—and thank God it did before too

many months dragged into years—when I realized that I held the rest of my life in my own hands, just as I always had, and that I still possessed the skill set and the strengths that had allowed me to succeed in the first place. My future could be bright as long as I personally ensured that it would be. It depended on no one other than me, and I began to see the power I held in that regard. I had become successful because I was a fine surgeon who loved his work and who was passionate about being the best surgeon he could be. Neither the end of my marriage nor the loss of my academic positions had altered those essential truths.

My recovery from my depression and the work of getting myself back in the saddle, so to speak, was helped immeasurably by the caring and supportive responses of many friends, colleagues, and even patients and their families. Although a few people in the Dallas medical community treated me rather coolly after my dismissal from Southwestern, the great majority of people I encountered on a daily basis made it very clear that I still held their friendship and respect. I remained on staff at Children's Medical Center and held operating privileges at Dallas's Baylor University Medical Center, and my work there continued successfully and without interruption.

My fellow craniofacial surgeons—several of whom had become dear friends over the seven or eight years since we had met—buoyed my spirits and kicked my butt in equal measure. Each man worked in a university setting himself and understood the constant headaches and significant impediments to progress that academic systems often imposed. Each also reminded me that although I was no longer a program administrator, I was indeed still a surgeon, one at work in a cutting-edge field, and that if I didn't want to be left behind I needed to refocus myself on surgery as intently as ever. I continued to be invited to meetings and symposia around the world, and journal editors made it clear that my contributions would remain welcome. In the spring of 1979, as had long been scheduled, I hosted in Dallas the annual meeting of the national Plastic Surgery Research Council, which I continued to chair.

As I worked to rebuild my life in a number of ways, I escaped the woebegone little apartment where I too often felt like a guy who'd recently been paroled. I purchased a cheery contemporary condominium that did its part in lifting my self-esteem; I visited my son, Ken, now a student at Texas A&M University, as often I could; and my daughter, Leigh, a high school student already, and I fell into a comfortable routine that allowed us to be with one another a couple of times each week. Shaaron and I began to reach the equilibrium and ongoing affection that everyone hopes for after a divorce. And enormously important, too, as I consciously navigated a comeback, was the fact that my patients continued to need me and the help I could offer them, just as I needed them to remind me of my truest purpose and responsibilities.

The particulars of my academic career had never been something to which my patients and their families paid attention, and I was gratified after my dismissal to discover that for families like the Couvalls, their continuing faith in me and their belief in the progress we were making with their daughter, Georgette, were far more important than any other consideration. The rapport we shared as we jointly agreed on each successive step in Georgette's transformation, and their unshakable resolve that I was the surgeon they wanted to lead the way, meant a great deal as the 1980s commenced, and both Georgette and I determined to remake ourselves in ways in which we could take pride.

The next step in Georgette's transformation was to reconstruct her nose. Because she had plenty of tissue on her forehead and between her eyebrows, I decided to shift some of that skin to her nasal area using what's known as a V-to-Y technique. This gave me more skin that I could use as cover for her new nose, but I also needed to create the foundation under the skin that would give it a natural shape. It was challenging work, but it was also just fundamental plastic surgery—creating over time a cartilaginous and bony framework made up of component parts that, on the exterior, offered the illusion of being entirely normal. In Georgette's case, I built that framework by taking cartilage from her ear, and bone and cartilage from her rib. But her nose, like everyone's, also needed to allow her to breathe, and I performed a variety of techniques on the inside of her nose to create functional nasal airways.

About a year after that procedure, it was time to move forward again, and now I took bone from her skull and split it into two equal pieces of half the original thickness. I returned one piece to her cranium, where it would heal and regain its strength; then I separated the split cranial bone graft into several pieces. With these new bone grafts I built up her cheeks to subtly give her face a more normal convex projection, balanced a portion of her jaw, and continued the reconstruction of her nose. I also refined the earlier work I'd done on her right eyelid and performed a lateral canthopexy—a procedure that strengthened her lateral can-thal tendon and surrounding structures to help maintain the normal position and relationship between her eyelid and her prosthetic eye. Georgette endured the long surgery remark-ably well, as had become her habit. And as I assessed her case in the months that followed, it seemed to me that we were about halfway to the point I hoped to reach one day. She now had a nose that was acceptable though certainly not perfect, and I had created a good eye socket where there had been none before. The proportions were a bit off, in my estimation, but we needed to let her grow and then reevalu-ate her. She'd come a long way; she was tough and resilient and she was maturing in remarkable ways—both physically and emotionally.

Perhaps in part because of her disabilities, Georgette was naturally a very giving and caring girl, and that attribute blossomed as we got to know each other better and better. She was almost always cheerful and was invariably optimis-tic about how each successive procedure would go. She had the endurance and determination of someone far older, and to put it simply, she made the very most of a life that was far from normal. Instead of being focused on friends and school and the simple joys of awakening to the world around her, Georgette's childhood was centered on doctor visits, hospi-tal stays, seemingly endless surgeries, pain, discomfort, and emotional challenges of every kind.

She shared with me the hurt she felt when other children would tease or taunt her, adding, "I especially hate it when people think I'm retarded just because of my face." Yet our biggest challenges are also often our greatest gifts, and today, as she nears forty, Georgette is a beautiful woman who devotes much of her time to offering counseling and other volunteer work to a number of organizations that care for children with cleft and craniofacial deformities. This is in addition to her full-time work at a company that provides bone- and blood-banking services.

She regularly talks to patients and parents who are just beginning to undergo what she did as a child, informing them about what to expect and assuring them that the long slog of surgeries is very much worth the ordeal. "I've been given so much," she told me when I spoke with her by telephone from her home outside Chicago recently. "I want to give back to all those other kids out there who have the problems I did. And I want people to look at kids with craniofacial problems and treat them like they're normal, not think of them as people who can't do anything, or can't speak for themselves. They need to know we're just like everyone else."

For years, I continued to perform surgeries at Baylor University Medical Center with the key members of the team I had assembled during my tenure at UT Southwestern, and I saw my private-practice patients there as well. It was a situation that allowed me both to sustain my focus on craniofacial surgery and patients like Georgette, and to build a thriving cosmetic surgery practice that offered me both satisfaction and substantial income for the first time in my career. I regularly performed the numerous operations that were popular at the time for the correction of aging—face-lifts, eyelids, nose and breast surgery, liposuction, and many others.

I did hand surgery and burn and trauma reconstruction as well, but my heart, energy, and vision were forever centered on craniofacial and cleft surgery, and I increasingly understood that reconstructive surgery and aesthetic surgery had much more in common than the public and even some surgeons tended to recognize. Many of the myriad techniques I became skilled at as I worked to improve the appearances of my cosmetic patients had direct applicability to reconstructive surgery. And very important, too, was the understanding I widely voiced to my colleagues that reconstructive surgery was inherently aesthetic surgery as well. It was a perspective that would eventually lead to the publication of *Techniques in Aesthetic Craniofacial Surgery*, a book that called for the marriage of craniofacial and aesthetic surgery in providing optimum outcomes and normal lives for these deformed children.

Unlike in orthopedic or abdominal surgery, for example—in which it really didn't matter how a hip replacement or gallbladder surgery looked as long as each procedure led to good function and good health—it *did* matter enormously how a new eye or nose looked for patients like Georgette. Her reconstructive surgery—and the surgeries of thousands of others—were *necessarily* aesthetic surgery as well.

Throughout the early eighties, my life and career slowly but nonetheless assuredly found their way onto an upward trajectory again. I had believed that my inability to play by the rules had destroyed my career, but it had only set it on a new course, and along the way I had learned a profound lesson that yielding to authority was absolutely necessary at times. In the aftermath of my divorce, I had worked hard to strengthen my relationship with my children and to spend as much quality time with them as I could, aware that early in their lives my focus on my work had kept me away from them far too often. Leigh sometimes traveled with me to meetings and conferences around the United States. She joined us on occasion when I was able to take my parents to Europe, Asia, and South America for the first time in their lives as part of my travels to attend meetings, consult, and perform surgeries. Those business and family trips remain particularly memorable.

Not long after I left Southwestern, I established a craniofacial fellowship, offering a year of close mentoring to young and very promising plastic surgeons from around the world. My first fellow was Yu-Ray Chen, an extremely bright and capable young surgeon from Taiwan who eventually returned to his country, where he and Dr. Sam Noordhoff developed a world-renowned plastic surgery and craniofacial hospital. I had met him when my team and I traveled to Taiwan in 1978 to perform the first craniofacial surgery ever offered there, and it's been my huge pleasure to return several times over the years as part of my international work.

In 1982, Ian Jackson, Ian Munro, Linton Whitaker, and I coedited the first *Atlas of Craniomaxillofacial Surgery*, an illustrated volume intended to help plastic surgeons around the world perform procedures with which they were not entirely familiar. A few years later, I joined my friend Dr. Janusz Bardach, who taught at the University of Iowa, in coauthoring *Surgical Techniques in Cleft Lip and Palate Surgery*, a book published first in English and later in Spanish. I had met Janusz, one of the most influential men in my life, in the early 1970s and invited him to Dallas, where he watched me do three cleft palate operations. The two of us bonded both as friends and as colleagues, and over time we jointly developed new procedures in cleft surgery, taught courses together, and lectured internationally as a two-person team, often "debating" each other and arguing opposing viewpoints to keep our presentations lively and engaging. Janusz was fun, very precise, and loved to play with ideas. We were known to delight our classroom audiences by challenging each other, often tongue-in-cheek.

Very quickly, our book became the bible for surgeons doing cleft lip and palate work around the world, and that was enormously gratifying. Children born with cleft lips and palates often present as some of the most tragically disfigured children we treat, yet surgeons can and routinely do transform their faces into virtual normalcy, leaving them with little more telltale sign of their former condition than a subtle vertical scar above their upper lip. From the time I

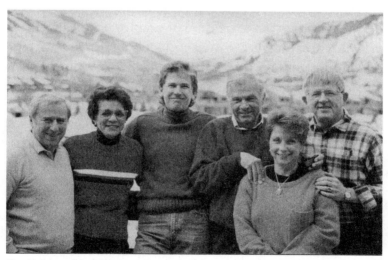

Dr. Salyer with friends and surgical associate (Janusz and Phyllis Bardach, Salyer, Hans Andrel, Rosalyn Patterson, Sam Noordhoff)

observed my first cleft surgery as a medical student in Kansas City, I've been moved by children born with this condition and by the profoundly successful ways in which it can be surgically treated. And it's been a source of pride for me not only to have performed thousands of successful cleft lip and palate surgeries during the course of my career but also to have helped legions of other surgeons improve their own techniques as they, in turn, have helped many thousands more.

Away from academia, I was able to create a very active and unique career in private practice, continuing to present, publish, do research, mentor, and teach, always emphasizing my clinical expertise in my private practice. But although I discovered that I could accomplish much that many people believed could only be actualized in an academic context, I wasn't satisfied with what I was achieving. In the best academic settings, it is the creation of teams of medical personnel who work together in dynamic and supportive ways over sustained periods of time in fully funded and well-equipped settings that produces the greatest advances and most stellar medical and surgical results.

I wanted to replicate that dedicated clinical and surgical center in the private health-care world, and to staff it with top-notch professionals who were invigorated by being part of a highly creative team. It seemed to me that such private centers could become commonplace not only for the treatment of craniofacial disorders but also in a wide variety of medical contexts. I began as early as 1979 to meet with hospital administrators throughout North Texas and beyond, hoping my vision would spark enthusiasm on their parts that would eventually lead to success. But although I had no difficulty convincing the people with whom I met of the need, no one could overcome the widespread fear that craniofacial surgery could never be profitable, nor was anyone willing to make the major financial commitment a stand-alone craniofacial center would require as its foundation.

But in 1985, I met Ira Korman, who was president and chief executive officer of Medical City Dallas Hospital, which at the time was operated by the health-care giant Humana. Although Ira had become a very successful upper-level executive, he wasn't a typical health-care administrator, at least as far as I was concerned. He held a PhD in psychology; he was a visionary who loved the challenge of turning bold concepts into reality; and I was certain, too, that being the father of a child with cerebral palsy helped him understand my passion for giving new lives to the young craniofacial patients under my care.

Ira's leadership had been responsible for Medical City Dallas's becoming one of the most successful facilities in the entire Humana empire; the hospital was earning profits of nearly fifty million dollars a year at the time, and besides having created renowned centers in adult cardiology, orthopedics, neurosciences, and diabetes, Ira was eager to accomplish more, especially for children. Instead of simply informing me that my dream was an impossible one—as I'd heard many times before—he listened intently over the course of many meetings as I described my vision of a craniofacial and pediatric neurosurgery center focused on academic research and state-of-the-art clinical care at Medical City.

The facility, as I envisioned it, would be staffed by key

members of the team of surgeons, physicians, and medical personnel with whom I currently worked in Dallas. Rosalyn Patterson, my scrub nurse at Children's Medical Center since my return to Dallas as a plastic surgeon, was an integral part of my professional life, someone who contributed significantly to the excellence I sought in the operating room and in all of my patient outcomes. Ed Genecov, a wonderful guy, was my primary orthodontist, someone who was very talented and who cared, as I did, about doing the very best work we possibly could. Trevor Mayberry was an otolaryngologist who provided our nose and throat care; Don Day, who at that time was the head of the Texas State Department of Genetics, was a pediatrician and a geneticist, and his regular consultations were invaluable. We lacked good speech pathology locally, but I had become close friends with Mary Anne Witzel, an internationally known speech pathologist from the Hospital for Sick Children in Toronto, and she had begun traveling to Dallas regularly to assist with cases that required her expertise. And Mike Lorfing, who had worked in the medical illustration department at UT Southwestern, now was eager to head our media department, which would be vitally important in creating high-quality still and video images of patients and surgeries, documentation that would be an integral part of the new center's research and educational programs.

But we would need to attract new members to the team as well, and at the top of my list was Ian Munro. By this time Ian, who pioneered craniofacial surgery in Canada at Toronto's Hospital for Sick Children, had created a very strong team of his own, but he had become disillusioned by changes in the Canadian health-care system, and I was confident that the creation of a center like the one I envisioned could entice him to move to Texas.

Pediatric neurosurgery was a subspecialty that had developed along a similar track and during the same era in which craniofacial surgery had advanced. The two subspecialties were closely allied in important ways, and I also envisioned bringing Dr. Derek Bruce, an internationally respected pediatric neurosurgeon at the Children's Hospital of Philadelphia, to Medical City to join us. Top-level pediatric neurosurgery had never been practiced in the Dallas area, and certainly not as part of a dedicated center that would serve children with both neurological and craniofacial disorders. Creation of a center that fully supported and sustained both subspecialties, staffed by some of the best medical professionals currently at work, would immediately make Medical City one of the foremost centers in the world for the treatment of children with challenging brain, head, and facial disorders.

I'll forever be grateful to Ira Korman for quickly grasping the scope of what I presented to him, the extraordinary level of care the center could offer, and the good we could do in the world. But he did more than simply begin to share my vision; he set about actualizing it with passion and utter determination. After many months of meetings, he, Ian Munro, Derek Bruce, and I boarded one of Humana's private jets and flew to Louisville, Kentucky, to meet with company founder and head David Jones and his board of directors. It was the final step toward reaching what had become our shared goal, and we were all very optimistic that it was about to be attained.

We met in the opulent boardroom at Humana's stunning

Michael Graves–designed headquarters in Louisville. David Jones, a lawyer and entrepreneur who was singularly responsible for Humana's enormous success, immediately took charge, and he was affable and engaging. Ira had created something special during his tenure at Medical City, Jones told us; the hospital was one he was already very proud of, and he was enthusiastic about how the center we proposed could make Medical City an even stronger hospital while at the same time contributing to Humana's meteoric financial growth.

We had arrived with an extensive pro forma outlining in

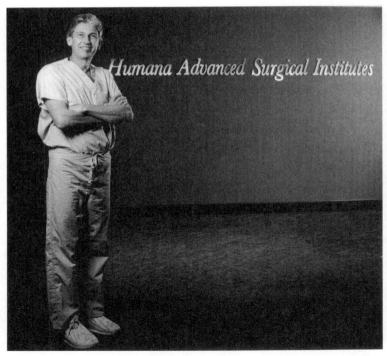

Dr. Salyer heralding the opening of the institute at Medical City Dallas

great detail every aspect of the state-of-the-art center, and surely Jones or some of his subordinates already had studied it—because instead of thanking us for coming and telling us they would get back to us, Jones rose at the end of the meeting, warmly shook our hands, and said, "Doctors, this is the part of my job that I love, and we're going to do great things together." He added that the new craniofacial institute at Medical City Dallas would receive twenty-eight million dollars in initial funding and Humana's wholehearted support—and with that we were under way.

By the time Alex Mather was born in nearby Fort Worth, the craniofacial institute was well established at the sprawling Medical City Dallas campus in the city's Hamilton Park neighborhood. Ira Korman had directed reconstruction at the hospital that created the finest clinical and surgical facilities in which I had ever worked, including two first-rate operating rooms dedicated specifically to craniofacial surgery, a third that was used solely for pediatric neurosurgery, a fully equipped research laboratory, state-of-the-art imaging facilities, a suite of examination rooms, an in-patient ward, and offices. Our primary staff totaled seventeen and included virtually everyone I had hoped to lure to Medical City—and to Texas—with this extraordinary opportunity. Fifty percent of our patients came from outside the state, and eventually we served children from all across the nation and seventy-five different countries, many of them indigent patients who received care virtually free of charge under the terms of our agreement with Humana.

The 1990s saw the institute emerge as perhaps the most important and certainly the busiest craniofacial facility in the world. There was so much work to do that I limited my practice to craniofacial and cleft lip and palate cases, and many of my patients—such as little Alex—presented the kinds of challenges that had pressed for the creation of the institute in the first place.

Alex was born at Harris Methodist Hospital in Fort Worth on January 31, 1992, with a cleft lip and palate, clubfeet, a scalp and skull defect that exposed his brain, strabismus—which prevents aligning the gaze of each eye and impedes binocular vision—and hydrocephalus, a condition in which fluid accumulates in the brain, enlarging the head and ultimately causing brain damage if the pressure of the fluid grows too great. His concert of disorders was so severe that the attending obstetrician suggested to his parents that they "just let nature take its course" and not attempt to close the gaping opening on top of their son's head. The obstetrician believed the combination of deformities was simply too much for the struggling infant to endure. But Alex's parents, Robert and Sherry Mather, disagreed. "God has a plan for Alex," Sherry insisted, and they wanted to give their son every possible opportunity to live.

When I first saw Alex in the spring of 1993, he had a very narrow, elongated skull, so pointed in the back that he couldn't lie on it. His thin skull bulged dramatically where his quickly growing brain pressed to escape its confines. The surgery that doctors had performed the day after his birth to close the opening on top of his head was inadequate and would need to be done again. He had a complete cleft of the lip and palate, plus a blockage in the back of his nose on the right side—a major concern because newborns are

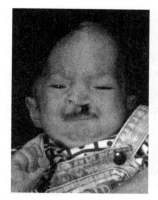 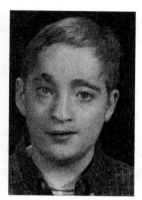

Alex before and after cranial reconstruction surgery

nose breathers and he would be at risk for airway problems. Alex's condition was dramatic, to say the least.

Adding to his tenuous situation, during that early surgery a ventricular peritoneal shunt had been inserted to drain the excess cerebrospinal fluid from his brain. A shunt placed that early in an infant's life can sometimes cause an abnormal collapse of the skull and induce craniosynostosis, a condition that leads to problems with normal brain and skull growth. It causes the pressure inside the head to decrease and the skull or facial bones to shift from a normal, symmetrical appearance—and that was what had happened to Alex. His head was grossly misshapen and appeared collapsed. From the outset, I was certain that Alex had been brought to the best place in the world for him, one that happened to be just forty miles from his parents' home. His clubfeet could be corrected by our team's pediatric orthopedic surgeon, but of foremost importance right then was to create new tissue, using tissue expanders, to replace the old scar tissue on his scalp and give his head adequate coverage to protect his brain. We took careful measurements across his skull to determine how much tissue was already available and usable and how much new, vascularized tissue would be needed. This was our first priority, and then we would begin to remodel his abnormally shaped skull.

I extensively planned the size of the expanders we would use and where I would place them under good tissue in Alex's scalp. The expanders were small balloons, in effect, that over time were filled with more and more saline solution, causing the skin to stretch and, ultimately, to grow. Once it was available, I would move the new tissue to replace a bald area about the size of a golf ball that could otherwise end up breaking down, ulcerating, and causing all kinds of problems.

There were other methods I could have used besides expanders to acquire needed tissue for Alex's head, but I believed this would be the best, simplest technique, even though it required multiple injections of saline over time. In Alex's case, we only had to sedate him lightly for those procedures, although some patients have to be put to sleep, and anesthesia always poses at least minimal risks that have to be taken into consideration.

At the same time I placed the expanders, I planned to operate on Alex's cleft lip and repair his nose. I had become adept enough at these two procedures that I had begun doing them during the same surgery, which few other plastic surgeons had the self-assurance to do. But by then I had twenty years of experience doing hundreds of these operations and following patients for years afterward to closely observe their progress. I was widely regarded as a cleft lip and palate expert, and I was always confident that I could create an aesthetically normal, functioning lip and nose with minimal deformity. By the time I began seeing Alex, I could perform these techniques with assurance. What *was* a new experience for me was to insert the predesigned tissue expanders in his scalp during the same surgery, but by now, too, long hours of incredibly intensive work had become entirely routine. Surgery and all its intensity were simply my job, and I loved it.

During this first operation, Alex was a perfect candidate for a technique I had developed primarily for the lip and nose. I took his existing nose apart, then created a new nose and lip, freeing the two bundles of abnormally displaced muscle on either side of the cleft and suturing them together to give his lip its proper shape and function. With the assistance of Eric Hubli, a terrific young surgeon who was my fellow at the time, in about two hours we were able to complete the primary lip and nose closure and insert the tissue expanders into both sides of Alex's head.

Within a few months, the swelling expanders had created new tissue on Alex's head. We removed them and created flaps of vascularized tissue with the new skin, which included hair-bearing tissue so he would have normal hair growth that would cover up the small residual scar that would be left from our incisions. That surgery was entirely successful, and Alex required no further treatment for his scalp. We could now proceed full steam ahead with the reshaping of his head.

Remodeling or reshaping a head is an integral, even fundamental element of craniofacial surgery. In my nearly fifty-year career, I've been involved with well over a thousand cranial vault remodeling cases, and the remodeling of the infant skull was pioneered by members of the International Craniofacial Club and a few others. It involves removing portions of the forehead, the frontal orbital rim around the eyes, and the temporal bones above the ears, as well as portions of the skull, when needed, to obtain as normal a skull shape as possible and still leave enough room for normal brain and facial function. When an infant like Alex has had a shunt placed to drain excess cerebrospinal fluid, in the remodeling process complications sometimes develop in keeping the dura, the tough lining that covers the brain, in contact with the skull, which is important for bone healing. Fluctuations in pressure in the brain's ventricles, which contain cerebrospinal fluid, can also adversely influence the remodeling and healing of the bone. Getting all this right can be a tricky dance at best, but I felt confident with Alex that we could achieve good results.

Alex's remodeling required two surgical stages, each of them dramatic. Working with team member Kenneth Shapiro, a fine pediatric neurosurgeon, in the first cranial vault surgery, I made an incision in the hairline, peeled down Alex's face, then removed two-thirds to three-quarters of the front of his skull, carefully dissecting around the defects and holes in his skull to allow the brain lining to achieve a more normal configuration. This was an extremely tedious operation requiring meticulous attention to detail as we performed the multitude of steps we had carefully planned. Next, we cut and reshaped each piece of bone so that when reinserted, the pieces—now a jigsaw puzzle—would expand the width of Alex's skull and shorten its length, creating the precise measurements we wanted for Alex's head and the positioning of his eyes. Alex once again proved to be a real

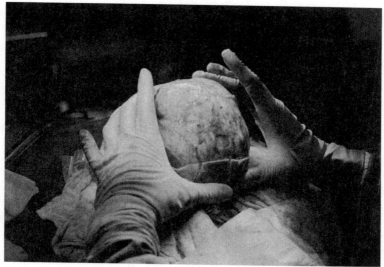

Dr. Salyer at work remodeling a child's skull

fighter; the surgery was remarkably successful, and we achieved the results we hoped for.

The team approach to these complex kinds of surgery has many advantages, particularly when it comes to administering as little anesthesia as possible. In Alex's case, for example, a few months later a single anesthesia allowed us to perform three new procedures at once: the rerotation of his clubfeet by Dr. Wally Bobechko, an internationally known orthopedic pediatric surgeon on our staff; placement of little grommet tubes deep in Alex's ears to drain fluid trapped by the tympanic membrane, performed by our staff otolaryngologist Tim Trone; and my correction of Alex's cleft palate.

Optimally, I like to repair a cleft palate early in the patient's first year, but Alex was almost a year old by the time we operated—a bit late but not worrisomely so.

The palate operation itself was one I helped develop. It involved the freeing of a group of muscles from either side of the mouth and suturing them together again in the back of the throat, a procedure, it seemed certain, that would ultimately allow Alex to speak normally.

As I operated, I was seated and Alex was positioned vertically and upside down, his head resting in the sterile area in my lap. This unusual arrangement allowed me to work deep inside his mouth and readily access the back of his throat, working very carefully to dissect out the muscle on each side, release it, then suture the complementary pieces together and carefully join them so there were no holes. Much later, we went back and grafted the area, using bone from Alex's hip to improve the alveolar gum region where the cleft had been, which would allow his teeth to erupt into the graft and create a strong dental arch. Today, it's difficult to tell that Alex ever had a cleft because he has normal teeth and both his upper lip and palate work well. It's pretty miraculous stuff.

Probably ten to twenty percent of the total number of patients I treat have strabismus—that is, their eyes appear to be looking in different directions and don't track normally. Alex suffered that disorder as well. He really had been born with many challenges, and I understood his parents' view that "God intended something important for him—and all you doctors and nurses are somehow part of the plan." At least with regard to his strabismus, the cure was simple and straightforward. Dr. David Stager, a Dallas-based pediatric ophthalmologist and expert in the field, briefly joined us in the operating room and in ten or fifteen minutes made a series of little incisions, shortening or lengthening one of the six muscles surrounding each eye as needed to align Alex's eyes and allow them to begin to move in concert.

All told, Alex was ultimately treated by a team that included twenty-five different specialists. Having all of us together at the institute served him and his medical outcome perfectly, allowing us to determine right from the outset who needed to see him and giving those of us who did the opportunity to brainstorm options. With Alex, we were dealing with many issues, and the ultimate plans of action and the surgeries themselves were far from simple. But we had the facility and the staff with which to address so many complicating factors—and of course each of us was seeing twenty or twenty-five patients like Alex in the clinic on any given day, each one in various stages of treatment.

This was the center and the level of care I had long ago envisioned—and it was enormously gratifying for me to have been able to shepherd it into existence, then observe what, in fact, we could accomplish. A little more than a decade before, I had sunk to the depths—and I could still summon the memory of that pain and despair. But it was wonderful to be able to quietly celebrate my *own* transformation and the actualization of a dream, an achievement that served thousands of children like Alex—and that served something deep inside me as well.

Although Alex's case was as difficult as any I ever encountered, it had an excellent outcome in the end. Alex had to endure fifteen surgeries and countless other procedures, but he went on to grow and develop virtually normally. Many kids with hydrocephalus have lifelong issues, but it's amazing how well some of them can do, and Alex is a good example. In spite of his ordeal, Alex's great attitude and positive outlook were evident early on. When he was five, his mother, Sherry, told me, a child pointed at him and asked, "Why does that kid have a crooked face?" Alex responded with complete assurance, "God made me that way."

Alex will soon be twenty-one. He has done well in school, he's retained his great sense of humor, and he's delightful to be around. His parents' early commitment to helping their son make the most of his challenges has been remarkable and no doubt has been a factor in his positive outlook and his triumph over the adversities that he was presented with as his life began. "Alex genuinely likes who he is," Sherry told me.

At the institute, I always did my best to remind my colleagues and the entirety of our team that although our focus each day was to create a new lip or reshape a patient's skull, our larger mission was to carve and give form to the totality of a young child's life.

Chapter Four

Two Faces

Nell Gozdowski remembers that when her daughter, Lindsey, was born, nurses immediately whisked her away in tense silence. "I only saw her precious little ear flattened against her head, but I had no idea what was going on," Nell recalls. "All I knew was that she didn't look right." And so began a long and difficult journey that Nell and Lindsey and their family would take together, one that ultimately brought them into my life, a voyage that might have daunted less courageous, determined individuals.

Lindsey was born with Goldenhar syndrome, a condition that generally means one side of the face is deformed or incompletely developed. In Lindsey's case, the right side of her face was severely affected, but the left side was normal. She had a very distorted and almost nonexistent right ear, and she was missing her right jaw, with no mandibular joint or cheekbone. She had a very undersize right eye socket and only a small, vestigial nonseeing eye with many little tumors—called dermoids—around and inside it.

In addition to these deformities, Lindsey also suffered from a heart valve defect, asthma, severe acid reflux, scoliosis, a full range of allergies, and most critically, apnea—

the sudden cessation of breathing, especially during sleep. Often, she would stop breathing completely during the night and then vomit all over herself as she gasped for air and her respiration revived. In the field of craniofacial surgery, we sometimes discuss a range of levels of difficulty when it comes to deformities and the particular challenges that interventions pose, and my personal scale consists of five levels. Lindsey was, without a doubt, a five on that scale and truly one of the most difficult cases of my career.

Before Lindsey became my patient, she and her family, who lived in the Toledo, Ohio, suburb of Sylvania, had already been through a great deal. Her first corrective surgery, which lasted sixteen hours, took place the summer she was two years old. In the days following, she developed a massive infection that destroyed the new bone her surgeon had grafted on the right side of her face and ate away what little original bone she had as well. During the next two years, relatively minor procedures developed into life-threatening situations. When her tonsils became so swollen that they obstructed her airway, an emergency tonsillectomy had to be performed, but only after she had been placed on a ventilator. Six months later, during a straightforward outpatient surgery, she went into respiratory and cardiac arrest, but the surgeon attending to her was able to revive her. When she was four, once more she suffered cardiac arrest during a simple visit to the dentist to have a cavity filled. Over the next five years, repeated efforts to surgically correct her deformities failed. And on one of these occasions, she contracted MRSA, a drug-resistant staph infection, which is always very serious and sometimes leads to death. MRSA is an organism that can lie dormant in tissue and return in future operations. Although that didn't happen in Lindsey's case, the infection not only ruined the results of the surgery, but also completely destroyed her small vestigial eye.

As Nell would later write, "When Lindsey became more aware of how she looked and how others perceived her, my husband and I felt that she deserved to have someone at least listen to her concerns and desires. She continued to have sleep-obstructive apnea, and when her surgeon told us he did not know how else to help Lindsey, we began yet another search for someone who could. And on Oprah Winfrey's television show, we discovered Dr. Salyer."

When I first met Lindsey, when she was nine, she had already endured *sixty* surgical procedures, but the results were extremely disappointing. She was beaten down and could barely speak. Both she and Nell literally begged me to help her. I was moved by her predicament—and touched by her spirit—and I wanted to do everything I possibly could. In my work, it's essential for me to establish mutual trust and instill the belief in my patients that we are making decisions jointly. I had received models of Lindsey's mandible and her skull in advance of that initial appointment, so I already had some understanding of the huge challenges that lay ahead of us. But I looked at Lindsey, and really connected with her, and I promised, "Yes, I can help you. Sure, I can help you."

From the time I first began to dream about the creation of a craniofacial institute, I imagined much more than simply the establishment of a state-of-the-art clinical practice. Perhaps in part because I once had presumed I'd spend my life in academic medicine, and certainly because I still understood how dynamic the combination of teaching, research, and clinical care can be, I wanted the institute to include vital elements of each of those three pursuits. And with the support of Ira Korman and Humana, we succeeded. Many years before, I had established a fellowship program in which I brought promising craniofacial surgeons to Dallas and mentored them for a year, and with the institute in place, people I considered the best and brightest young surgeons in the world now were all the more eager to come to Dallas to learn and further develop their skills. I had enlisted a stellar team to join me beginning in 1986, and together we offered what I was convinced was one of the finest clinical and surgical craniofacial practices in the world at the time. And we were able to make a commitment to research as well—both basic research and translational research, whose goal is to quickly and efficiently apply the basic research findings to meaningful health outcomes for patients.

Ira Korman oversaw the renovation of the basement of our building at Medical City into both operating rooms and laboratories, with Humana providing initial financial support for the research, which we later augmented with governmental and foundation grants. We hired three PhD scientists whose primary interest was in basic research problems related to craniofacial surgery and neurosurgery, and soon we were bringing patient-specific issues to them with hopes that they could offer both nonsurgical perspectives and insights—which they regularly and very valuably did—as well as investigate issues for which none of us yet had answers.

Initially Ian Munro, Derek Bruce, and I—the three surgeons on our team—saw our own patients and brought in the others for consultation when we thought they could be of specific help. My practice was the largest and busiest at the beginning because I had become well known in Dallas during the preceding two decades. Many Canadian patients followed Dr. Munro to Dallas, immediately making us an institute whose reach extended beyond US borders. With the international reputation as a pediatric neurosurgeon that Dr. Bruce had built in Philadelphia, he soon was attracting young patients from around the world who suffered difficult-to-treat brain tumors—many of which he increasingly removed using craniofacial surgery techniques and entry points, allowing easier access to the tumors through transfacial routes. Each of us was able to make many of these kinds of advancements and improvements specifically because we were able to learn so much from each other and from everyone on the institute team.

A nucleus of staff specialists spent their time seeing our patients clinically and offering diagnoses and treatment plans. John Kolar, a physical anthropologist whom Ian had known in Toronto and greatly admired, played a vital role in taking detailed and complex measurements of all of our patients pre- and postoperatively. He distinguished himself as a clinical anthropologist and ultimately published a book on craniofacial measurement, wrote a newsletter and numerous articles, and gave presentations on behalf of the institute at meetings worldwide.

Speech pathologist Judy Tobe later joined Mary Anne Witzel, giving us outstanding practitioners in that area. Derek Bruce lured his friend and colleague Ken Shapiro from New York City, where he had been a professor of neurosurgery at Montefiore Medical Center, and Ken was a wonderful addition to the team. And from just across town,

Grady Crosland, a pediatric anesthesiologist who had been at Children's Medical Center of Dallas, joined us as well. A superb anesthesiologist and a great guy, Grady would ultimately join me in performing more than five thousand surgeries, and to this day, there is no one in the world I would rather have monitoring my patients as I operate on them.

Together with orthodontist Ed Genecov, ENT surgeon Trevor Mayberry, pediatric geneticist Don Day, my indispensable scrub nurse Rosalyn Patterson, and many others, we were able to offer better and more comprehensive care than had ever been available anywhere in the world. And it was only because of their expertise, their dedication, and the spiritual belief each of them held in the importance of their work that, in the end, I was able to keep my promise to Lindsey, and to many other patients like her.

From the beginning of my relationship with Lindsey and her parents—and all of us truly did create strong bonds with each other—I knew there was something very special about

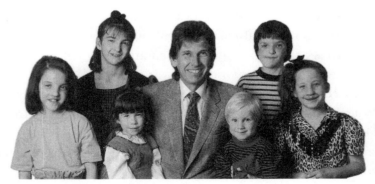

Dr. Salyer with former patients

her. As I've written, hundreds of the young people with facial deformities whom I've met over the years have created remarkable lives out of the challenges they have had to confront. Still, Lindsey stands out as someone whom I hold in the very highest regard. Few of my patients have had to deal with as many physical challenges as Lindsey, and very few possess her valiantly indomitable spirit.

"I don't really see myself as different from anyone else," she wrote in a letter to me a number of years ago.

I don't want anyone else to see me as different either, because I am not. I want to get in trouble when I deserve it, just like everyone else. I want to be recognized for the things I do well when I have earned recognition. I don't want to be remembered in school or by friends just as the person who had a lot of surgeries....However, most people do judge a person by their appearance. They try to break this habit, but still find themselves continuously judging others. They may not understand how much it hurts someone's feelings until it happens to them....I want people to remember me for who I am, not what I look like. I'm Lindsey, and I love social studies and hanging out with my friends. I dream about becoming a doctor and helping patients like all of you have helped me. If I could change just one thing, I wouldn't change how I look. I'd change how people look at me.

It was my job to change the way Lindsey looked, of course, and even more importantly, to help her eat, breathe, and sleep as normally as possible and eventually bring her seemingly endless series of surgeries to a successful close. She and her parents were terrifically supportive as we planned a multistep, many-surgery approach to meeting our collective goals. Lindsey had grown much more optimistic in the months since we had met, and I reminded her often that I was depending on her to keep a positive attitude and set intentions for success. Lindsey's mother, Nell, had appeared very proactive about her daughter's care when I first met her, and by now she was completely engaged, believing that at last we would succeed, calling me frequently to discuss what should or shouldn't be done, what we should try, and whether she should see anyone else in addition to me and my colleagues at the institute. Nell was committed to getting top results—and I was delighted.

The first surgery I performed on Lindsey was a big one—extensive, long, and dramatic. As a routine but critical first step, we would need to intubate her, inserting a tube down her throat and trachea and into her lungs so her breathing could be carefully monitored and controlled during

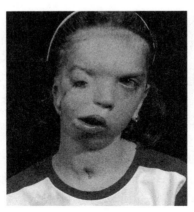

Lindsey at the time Dr. Salyer met her

the many hours the surgery would last. But her deformed jawbone, together with the scar tissue that had fused her mandibular joint, left her unable to completely open her mouth. Her airway was compromised, and the problem was exacerbated by the tracheostomies she'd needed when she came close to death during those two earlier crises. Dr. Jim Rothschiller, a top pediatric anesthesiologist at Medical City, had intubated Lindsey in preparation for several previous surgeries. He was the one person the family had confidence in and who had proven capable of intubating Lindsey successfully—and we were absolutely committed to success. So from the outset, we knew that whenever Lindsey needed to be put to sleep, the first order of business would be to make sure Jim was her anesthesiologist.

I knew, too, that continuity of care would be important at every stage, and I wanted Dr. Raul Barceló—a native of Mexico who initially had come to Dallas as one of my craniofacial fellows and by now had joined us at the institute—to be my primary assisting surgeon each time we operated on Lindsey. Lindsey loved Raul's smooth Latin style and readily connected with him. We would be performing a number of surgeries on this brave little girl, including some very advanced and innovative procedures, and I would need people assisting me like Raul and my steadfast scrub nurse Jenna, with whom I had worked seamlessly and efficiently for so many years and with whom I knew I could do my very best work.

The primary goal of the first surgery was to remodel the skeletal structure of the right side of Lindsey's face. Her vestigial eye and some of the orbital bone surrounding it had been lost because of her earlier infection, and we needed to create a larger, stronger eye socket in which to place a prosthetic eye. To achieve this, I took a large piece of cranial bone from above her forehead, split it into two pieces, and returned half to its original position. I carved the other piece into the shape of the bone I needed, and it became part of the new eye socket. Working intracranially to protect her brain, I cut her eye socket out as a box, moved it up and in, and expanded it so it could hold an artificial eye after it had healed. The final result was slightly smaller than the socket on her left side, but that was acceptable, particularly because I was successful in moving it into alignment with the left. It was a major task, one that required me to fill in spaces around the orbit with bone grafts but also use bone grafts to create a new zygomatic (cheek) bone to match the one on her left side.

Now that we had moved her eye socket to a better position

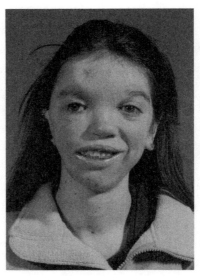

Lindsey after her first operation with Dr. Salyer

and supported it with bone grafts and cheekbone, we were able to place Lindsey's new prosthetic eye, which made a dramatic difference in her upper face. The eye was not quite full-size because the orbit was necessarily a bit smaller than her left one, nor did she have the musculature that would have allowed her prosthesis to move like a normal eye; but given the point from which we had started, it was a significant step forward.

The best thing about the first surgery was that it provided Lindsey and her parents with a taste of success. They had suffered so many defeats in the years before that this was not just a meaningful transformation but also a demonstration that something dramatic could indeed be accomplished. I always want patients like Lindsey to see real change early in the process, which engenders their hope and confidence that we can accomplish much more.

Next, we needed to surgically free Lindsey's frozen mandibular joint, which was comparatively simple. Once that was done, we were able to begin a series of operations designed to give Lindsey a serviceable right jaw using a remarkable technique called distraction. This was a surgical procedure that had been used for some time to produce new bone growth and thereby lengthen the bones of the arms and legs, but at the time, distraction was just beginning to be used in craniofacial surgery—and it was as new to me as it was to Lindsey.

At its most basic, the procedure is one in which a surgeon severs the mandible, or lower jawbone, on both sides of the face. The surgeon then anchors a metal appliance to the separated bones, one that incorporates a screw mechanism that, when turned little by little each day over a period of weeks, expands the gap between the two pieces of bone. New bone rapidly forms as the gap widens. Once the desired length is achieved, the turning stops and the device is left in place until the bone is consolidated.

Distractors can be placed internally or externally, depending on a variety of circumstances. In Lindsey's case, we opted to use external hardware, and unlike with most patients, we only needed to create new bone on the right side of her jaw because her left side had developed normally. It was a long and taxing process for her, one that required distraction of her maxilla simultaneously over time, creating new bone to move her upper and lower jawbones forward, millimeter by millimeter, day by day, into a more normal position. At each stage, we worked to get the upper and lower jaws to match and, for the first time in her life, give her a symmetrical face.

For a young girl who longed to look normal, it was a particularly tough time. She was forced throughout that period to wear a framework of stainless steel hardware on her face and head, including a so-called rigid halo that circled her skull for her upper jaw distraction. But Lindsey, bless her heart, understood that we could only reach our collective goals if we were patient, and she knew that acquiring a face that allowed her to blend in with her classmates at school would necessitate dozens of surgeries as well as standing out *more*, not less, for longer than any of us would have liked. She understood, too, that the work we were doing on her jaw wasn't just for looks; it was to address—and end, we hoped—the life-threatening sleep apnea that had plagued her so long.

In the midst of it all, Lindsey's parents made sure her life was as fulfilling as possible—and I applauded them for their dedication. Back home in suburban Toledo, she took gymnastics and swimming lessons; she joined a girls' soccer league; she tried for and got a role in a junior opera production, sang karaoke and a solo in a school Christmas program—even served as the auctioneer at a Make-A-Wish Foundation fund-raiser. I still have a copy of the letter Lindsey's mom sent me describing how remarkably her daughter was coping. "Lindsey has developed an intuition of knowing how to handle people who stare at her," she wrote.

> She realizes that people are just naturally curious and has learned to talk with people who can't take their eyes off her. She just talks to them about everyday life to make them more comfortable and, if they have questions about her appearance, she answers them. Also, Lindsey has quite a sense of humor. In fact, prior to the first surgery you performed on her, she informed her classmates that she was going to Dallas to get breast enlargements!

Over a period of about four years, my team and I succeeded in creating a foundation of facial bone for Lindsey that she hadn't had before. We used distraction techniques to allow her to grow new bone of her own throughout the right side of her face, aligning upper and lower jaws that once had been markedly deficient and displaced. Our creation of a bony eye socket out of cranium bone for her right eye, plus a number of other procedures, were major successes. After her facial skeleton was in place, I did some soft-tissue corrections that were helpful, and Raul Barceló has continued to make improvements around her eyes and has created a very normal right ear for her as well.

Lindsey's nineteen years old now, and she and I remain in close touch, although I seldom see her. She reminds me of so many other children—now adults—I've known through the years who have had to contend with truly severe deformities. In the beginning, they are really desperate; they can't see any way to escape their situation. But then, all of a sudden, there *is* real change. It's unmistakable; their face *is* more normal, they begin to blossom in wonderful ways, and their individual personalities emerge. This happened quite terrifically with Lindsey.

When we first met, she and her parents were adamant that they wanted her appearance to be the best it could be, and even though hers is one of the most difficult cases I've taken on, we've been able to make significant improvements. And with the help of Dr. Eduardo Rodriguez, a renowned microsurgeon at the University of Maryland

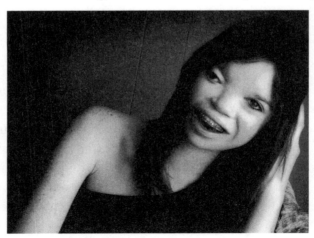

Lindsey today after her surgeries

Medical Center who recently performed the world's most extensive whole-face transplant to date, Lindsey has a newly reconstructed temporal mandibular joint and she looks terrific. She has become a young adult; she's graduated from high school and is heading to college. She's set her sights on becoming a craniofacial surgeon one day, and it's difficult for me to describe how touched I am that that is her goal. She has the intelligence, motivation, stamina, and patience to succeed, and I believe she will. Lindsey reminds me a bit of myself at her age in her determination to contribute and to do so by becoming a physician, and I've shared with her something of a secret that I hope will help minimize any worries she might have about her limitations.

When I was a youngster, I enjoyed hunting with my father and grandfather. But even though I'm right-handed, I couldn't see well when I sighted a rifle using my right eye, so I started shooting left-handed, using my left eye. When my dad decided it would be a good idea to have my eyes checked, an ophthalmologic examination revealed that I had severe amblyopia with dramatically suppressed vision in my right eye. For long stretches, I wore a patch on my good left eye to try to stimulate the vision in my right eye, and I regularly did a variety of exercises to build it up. But it was too late.

Throughout the rest of my life, most of my vision has come from my left eye. That means that during all the surgery I've performed over nearly fifty years, I've lacked the fine three-dimensional vision that requires two good eyes. Yet that early disability didn't prevent me from becoming a fine surgeon, and neither will having just a single eye prevent Lindsey from becoming an outstanding surgeon—*if* she ultimately decides it's the right career for her. I love this girl as if she were my own daughter, and just as any father would affirm, I'm convinced she can do anything she sets her heart on.

Our creation of the best plan of care for complex cases like Lindsey's was greatly assisted by our commitment to staying in close communication with one another and ensuring that all of us at the institute kept abreast of the most cutting-edge developments in our respective fields. Toward that end, we all gathered regularly to discuss patients and treatment options for them, and we held frequent teaching conferences as well. Ian Munro and I took turns leading a weekly craniofacial conference, attended by the entire craniofacial team, and Ed Genecov and I led a reconstructive orthodontics conference as well—my early-life interest in dentistry still with me after many decades. Patients like Lindsey were the focus of lively, stimulating gatherings at which collective brainstorming and the open expression of differing perspectives and approaches often led to innovative plans for treatment we might otherwise have overlooked or never envisioned. The gatherings were informal yet rigorous, and I always enjoyed and respected the ways we were able to challenge one another and compete intellectually yet remain committed to the teamwork we all believed in so strongly.

Vital members of our team were neuroradiologist Crys Sory and his group of Dallas-based pediatric neuroradiologists, who provided superb imaging and diagnostics, without which reaching an accurate preoperative understanding of a patient's internal anatomy and condition would have been very difficult. Initially, they—and we—relied on CT scans and MRIs to give us the information we needed, imaging technology that produced two-dimensional "slices" of the inside of a skull, for example, from neck to crown. When the slices were displayed side by side, it was relatively easy to envision the interior of the skull in three dimensions.

But medical imaging took great leaps forward with computer software that made 3-D images out of the serial slices, as well as the development of stereolithography in the late 1980s, a process that now could create models of skulls, brains, vascular networks, or anything inside the body that we needed to visualize and understand in great detail. Using digital information provided by CT scans, a stereolithography machine can quickly and accurately create a model by building a single layer, just half a millimeter thick, out of liquid resin. With each successive layer, a resin-filled blade sweeps across the cross section at the model's base, recoating it with fresh material whose proper pattern is traced by a laser. The process is repeated hundreds of times until a precise life-size model is complete. Once immersed in a chemical bath to clean away excess resin, then cured in an ultraviolet oven, the model is ready.

Our ability, beginning in about 1990, to take that model, hold it in our hands, turn it, and study it from dozens of angles was an extraordinary advance in safety, teaching, and clinical care. Once these models became available, I didn't need to order a model or models for all my patients before surgery, but I certainly did with major cases like Lindsey's; and an additional benefit was that, unlike two-dimensional imaging, which was often quite difficult for patients to make sense of, 3-D models were excellent tools to have at hand in consultation with the patients and families as we discussed a proposed surgical treatment.

We were also greatly assisted by the medical illustrator on our team, who would make a life-size photographic print of a patient, then meticulously draw the patient's face as we imagined it corrected. Next, the drawing was overlaid on the patient's photograph, allowing the illustrator to take fine and precise measurements of the amount of movement of the soft tissues that would be necessary to achieve an attractive and balanced face. We would use those drawings in combination with CT and MRI data, as well as those remarkable three-dimensional resin models, at our weekly craniofacial conference. Collectively they supplied incredibly detailed and sophisticated images that allowed all of us—craniofacial surgeons, speech pathologists, neurosurgeons, orthodontists, anthropologists, medical illustrators, otolaryngologists, pediatricians, geneticists, radiologists, and other appropriate specialists—to rapidly grasp the complexities of a given patient's conditions as a prelude to seeking consensus on a plan of attack.

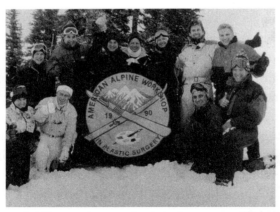

Dr. Salyer with fellow surgeons at the second American Alpine Workshop in 1991

Along the way, we were ably assisted by nursing, computer, and clerical employees as well, and each of the several lead surgeons oversaw a staff of between twenty and thirty support personnel. The institute became a hive of activity throughout each day—a setting that was a thrill for me to walk into each morning. Of course, the children we were serving were part of the high-energy scene in ever increasing numbers as well. They were the reason we were there, after all.

By the mid-1990s, our patient load was growing at a fast enough pace that we were able to add to the team Dr. Wally Bobechko, a pediatric orthopedic surgeon from the Hospital for Sick Children in Toronto with an international reputation in scoliosis. Working in concert, we created a bona fide academic center for craniofacial and pediatric neurosurgery in a nonacademic private hospital—a rare achievement. It was wonderful to actualize the dream that had motivated me for so long, and to see and be part of its great success.

Luke Rinehart is a remarkable young man from Oregon who from birth has also faced the devastating facial abnormalities of Goldenhar syndrome, but he and Lindsey have responded to their challenges in differing ways—a fact that highlights for me the reality that every patient is unique and that, ideally, each of us responds to the trials life presents us in the individual ways that serve us best.

Although both Lindsey and Luke have met their personal disabilities with an inspiring optimism and dignity, Luke has shied away from some surgeries and procedures that might have made greater improvements in his physical appearance, simply accepting the way he looks as part of the totality of who he is. The fact that he is a male in a culture that puts less pressure on men and boys than it does on women to meet a societal definition of beauty certainly played a role in shaping Luke's attitudes about his face. And the rural, outdoor lifestyle he has cherished since early childhood also has helped him focus on his physical and social abilities more than his physical appearance.

Yet Luke and Lindsey—different in many ways—share the wonderful ability not simply to accept their disfiguring medical condition but, at least in part, to become remarkable people *because* of it. And, too, they share a terrific sense of humor and a joie de vivre that is infectious. Luke's passions are skiing, hiking and climbing, team sports, rock music, and wildlife conservation, and as a proud native of Oregon—growing up in Crater Lake National Park, where his father is a ranger—he's never been able to resist ribbing me about my adopted state of Texas. "Hey, I'm Luke," he wrote a few years ago in a wonderful letter of support to kids who are currently undergoing the many surgeries he did as a child. "I'm twenty-one years old. I've been coming to Dallas to see Dr. Salyer since I was eighteen months old. And yeah, it's an okay place—if you like the heat, the Dallas Cowboys, and hospitals!"

As he explained in his letter, he hoped what he had to say would help others cope with their own facial disfigurements: "Goldenhar syndrome is what I have, but it is not who I am. It stops me from doing nothing."

Like Lindsey, Luke was born with one side of his face severely underdeveloped and malformed, but in his case it was his left side. He, too, had a smaller eye and orbit than on his normal-appearing side, and a tiny vestigial ear that

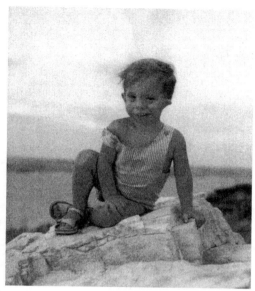

Luke Rinehart as a young boy, before surgery

needed reconstruction. He was missing much of his lower jawbone, and his upper and lower jaws did not meet properly. As Luke mentioned in his letter, I first met him when he was eighteen months old, and a few months later we began his treatment with a common strabismus surgery, an operation on the extraocular muscles of his left eye to correct its misalignment. A year later, I performed a rib graft, using the bone from his chest to build the skeletal structure for a more normal lower jaw.

Luke was seven when I referred him to Dr. Burt Brent in the San Francisco area, who was the best in the world at that time at reconstructing malformed or underdeveloped ears. Dr. Brent's approach is to create a whole new ear by taking rib cartilage and carving it into a new ear framework, then draping normal skin over it. Other common approaches employ a prosthetic frame under the normal skin or an entirely prosthetic ear attached via an implanted titanium hinge. The several procedures ultimately give patients a remarkably normal-appearing external ear, but the underdevelopment of the ear canal and middle ear structures, as well as the hearing loss that normally accompanies ear deformities, is quite difficult to treat surgically. Luke had very little hearing on his left side, and Dr. Brent was unable to change that.

Luke was nine when he and his parents came back to me, and it was immediately very clear that he was becoming a lively, outgoing boy who really enjoyed his life. Luke told me, "I love soccer, fishing, skiing, swimming—anything outdoors. I'm going to be a park ranger like my dad when I grow up." Apart from having an abnormal face, he was a boy like any other, who had lots of friends, was curious and energetic, and no doubt occasionally needed a little discipline. Unlike most nine-year-old patients—who by that age are old enough that they have become very aware of their conditions—Luke didn't let his deformity truly bother him. Nor were his parents hyperconcerned about how he looked or the likelihood that he would be ridiculed or discriminated against sometime in the future. I remember his mother, Deborah, describing his deformity as only "a moderate imperfection," and she assured me that it had just a minimal effect on his overall quality of life. The family simply incorporated Luke's condition into their normal lives and carried on.

During that visit, I operated on Luke's upper jaw to try to better align it with his lower jaw for proper closure. But my efforts to obtain optimum results were hampered because he was unable to have orthodontic treatments in the very rural area where he lived, and perfect alignment of his teeth was never achieved. But he was fine, he assured me. He was pleased with the degree of success we'd achieved, and so were his mom and dad.

A year later, I implanted external distraction devices on both sides of his lower jaw, and over the course of about four months we achieved two and a half centimeters of new bone growth—an excellent result. I was content with the shape his jaw was assuming as he entered his teenage years.

Luke was twenty before I saw him again in April 2003, and I was as drawn to him as I had been when he was young. He was self-confident and engaging and, most of all, happy. He liked his life—and his face—but he'd matured enough that for the first time I could tell that he wouldn't mind looking even better. That spring, I performed a major Le Fort I surgery, moving his whole midface forward. That surgery, too, was very successful, and a few months later, Luke announced he'd had enough. I discussed with him a variety of additional procedures that I felt certain would lead to overall improvement, but now a young adult—and working on a trail crew in the national park where he'd grown up—he opted against them. Over the course of the previous eighteen years, we had employed cranial bone grafts, rib grafts, dermal grafts, bilateral mandible distractions, and a number of other procedures to reshape his face. And although vestiges of his Goldenhar syndrome certainly remained, I was sanguine about the outcome, not because it was perfect or what it might have been, but because Luke himself was satisfied, and that was what mattered most.

Along the way, and with his parents' blessing, he had

declined surgeries when they would have interfered with playing football—yes, he played football in middle school and throughout high school! And he had been adamant about not wanting to have his teeth or jaws wired or to have any other procedure that would hold him back or slow him down. He had become one of the most well-adjusted and positive young men I've ever met—whether disabled or not—and I was grateful for the lesson he taught me. It was the truth that achieving my own idea of perfection for a patient is far less important than getting us to a point and an appearance that is exactly right for him or her.

"Be strong. Smile," Luke continued in his letter to my future patients:

> Don't limit yourself. I find my defect to be a fine way to meet challenges that otherwise would not be challenging. I see it as an opportunity to be unique in a unique way. If you ever need advice or a question answered, feel free to look up some of us old veterans. And if you find me in the middle of the mosh pit at a rock concert, just don't tell Dr. Salyer. Catchya on the flip side, Luke.

Luke is about a decade older than Lindsey, and living two thousand miles apart, they have never met, although through the stories I've shared, they know of each other. I certainly wouldn't presume to do any matchmaking, and I'm sure I think of them at the same time so often simply because they both share the challenges of Goldenhar's. But more than that, they share something that seems to me to be the pinnacle of the human spirit, a priceless ability

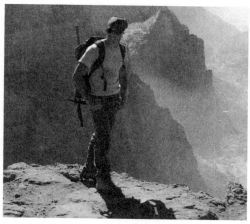

Luke Rinehart as an adult

to find joy in living when others of us so often struggle to do so. Luke is remarkable and inspiring, and will, I know, go on to live a full and very meaningful life. As will Lindsey, because, as she sometimes likes to say with a broad smile, "I'm so much more than just a pretty face."

Chapter Five

The Dogaru Girls

From 1969 to 2006, I performed over sixteen thousand operations in Dallas, including more than five thousand craniofacial cases and more than five thousand cleft lip and palate cases. Beginning in 1986, when we created the institute, I limited my practice to those two types of reconstructive surgery, no longer performing aesthetic or cosmetic surgery, simply because I was so busy doing what I loved best.

At the institute, my work settled into a wonderful rhythm of taking on both routine and very challenging cases, and it became a career I wouldn't have dared to dream of back when I was fired a decade before. About thirty percent of the patients we treated at the institute were funded by Medicaid or were so-called free-indigent patients from whom we received few or no fees because they didn't have the ability to pay. It felt great to be able to offer the care and treatment we did to so many children who otherwise would have been turned away—many of whom *had* been turned away before they came to us. And in many ways, we also significantly influenced the way cranio-facial surgery was practiced around the world.

We discovered, for example, that it isn't necessary to shave a patient's head before making an incision above the hairline in order to avoid infection—an innovation that was minor but that meant a great deal to many patients and their parents. When we began, the use of pressure dressings and drainage tubes that were inserted postoperatively was the norm. But we found that spinal fluid drainage simply isn't necessary as a matter of course and that pressure dressings on incisions and wounds are seldom helpful.

As our surgical techniques became more efficient, the length of our patients' hospitalizations decreased and their complications were minimized. Young patients normally spent only a single day in the pediatric intensive care unit after major intracranial surgeries—something that would have been unheard of ten years before. We began to discharge patients as soon as the swelling around their eyes subsided and they could see—normally after just three to five days. Our techniques for taking iliac cancellous bone grafts from the hips of our cleft patients improved so much that they could walk out of the hospital and go home the next day with little or no pain or other complications.

We developed techniques as simple as making initial incisions in the hairline in a zigzag pattern, which became standard around the world, allowing the patient's hair to obscure the scar and eliminating the harsh straight-line incision and the attendant stigma of having had surgery. And in a far more dramatic way, we were able to prove how amazingly well a child can recover from having his or her head and skull opened and brain exposed for major craniofacial and/ or pediatric neurosurgical care. Children wake up from the surgery with very minimal disability, allowing them to proceed with renewed confidence and, often, with a very normal life. This achievement made it possible for us to resolve craniosynostosis—which often causes a dramatically mis-shapen skull when a young patient's cranial sutures fuse prematurely—by cutting the cranium into a number of pieces and remodeling the entire cranial vault. In treating cranio-synostosis and a variety of related disorders with whole-skull remodeling, we proved that even patients with the most heart-breakingly disfigured heads could become normal-looking.

It was extraordinary good fortune for all of us at the institute to be present at such an exciting moment in recon-structive medicine. We had the privilege and the challenge of helping to develop an entirely new surgical subspecialty—and we made the most of it—but our biggest reward was the transformation of thousands of children and their lives.

My personal good fortune at Medical City Dallas continued in the sweltering summer of 1987 when a beautiful young

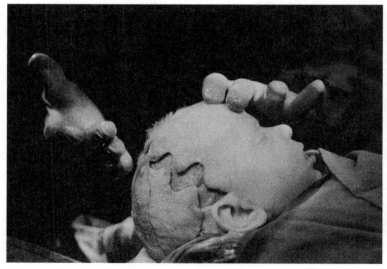

A surgical approach to the reconstruction of the face and skull

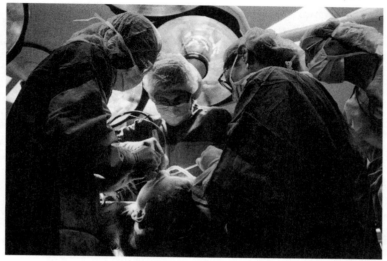

Dr. Salyer in the operating room

woman named Luci Lara applied for a clerical job and was hired. Born in the city of Monterrey in Mexico, Luci had grown up in Dallas, and her interest in health and wellness sprang naturally from the fact that for many generations women in her family had been *curanderas*, folk healers. Luci possessed a *curandera*'s healing gifts, it was clear to me as I began to get to know her. It was great to have her join us, and after a number of months, she and I began to date. Our relationship blossomed rather quickly into a profoundly meaningful one, and she brought wonderful balance to my life—introducing me to meditation, a personal spirituality I hadn't known before, and a number of alternative healing modalities, both ancient and modern, that opened my eyes and challenged me to consider many aspects of my profession in vital new ways. We began to live together in 1988 and were married in Telluride, Colorado, where we built a second home, in 1994.

From the outset of our relationship, Luci became a wonderful traveling companion. Both of us love the adventures and discoveries of travel, and neither of us is unduly put off by travel's intrinsic aggravations and complications. We made our first medical trip together in 1989, traveling to Moscow, where I had been invited to introduce craniofacial surgery to surgeons at the city's Burdenko Neurosurgery Institute, named after its founder, Nikolay Burdenko, the father of Soviet-era neurosurgery. The Soviets had become widely renowned for the quality of their neurosurgery during the twentieth century, but craniofacial surgery was entirely new to them.

We journeyed to Moscow just weeks after the Berlin Wall fell; the end of the Soviet empire had gone from unthinkable to entirely conceivable in a very short time. The Soviet economy was in terrible shape, and the state-owned medical infrastructure throughout the country fared little better. Our host, Professor Alexander Konovalov, then head of the institute and the foremost neurosurgeon in the Soviet Union, greeted us warmly at our hotel on our arrival and was quick to confess that in addition to its poor facilities, "only few of fifty neurosurgeons on Burdenko staff are very good."

Walking into the drab, hulking building was like stepping back in medicine fifty years or more. A strange and unpleasant odor—one very different from the normal smell of a hospital—hung in the air, the lighting was poor, and electricity was so undependable that surgical instruments had to be powered by pressurized gas. I remember people going about their duties rather joylessly, and I couldn't blame them.

My initial invitation to travel to Moscow had come from a Russian research scientist at the National Institutes of Health in Washington who was the father of a craniosynostosis patient on whom I had operated. Father and son had returned to the Soviet Union some time before, and the father had lauded my talents to Dr. Konovalov and had shared with him my desire to help spread the practice of high-quality craniofacial surgery. Our plan was to meet Konovalov and his top surgeons and discuss whether the time was right to introduce them to craniofacial surgery. We also wanted to consult with a number of patients to determine whether it might make sense to return later with a whole team for surgeries on a number of very needy children.

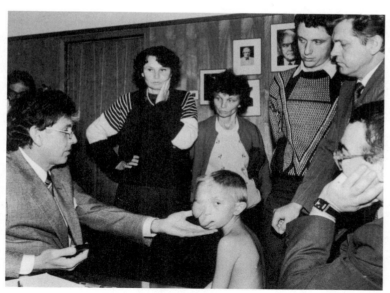

Russian patients with neurofibromatosis

I'll never forget the moment when, in the midst of a surgery—with the patient's head open and brain exposed—I glanced up and seemed to see something that I couldn't possibly be seeing. A high ledge encircled the room near the ceiling, and sitting on it rather magisterially and now unmistakably was a cat, which calmly observed the flurry of activity below.

"Yes, cat," Dr. Konovalov said when he saw the look of astonishment my surgical mask couldn't hide. Then he explained how a cat had indeed found its way into an operating room at this prestigious facility. "We have cats because we also have rats. And mice. Cats are on staff, you could say." It made some sense, I had to admit; better to have a cat in an operating room than a rat. And our overall experience

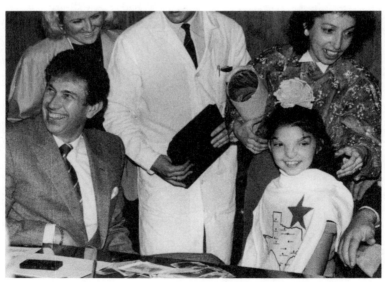

Dr. Salyer with a Russian patient in Moscow

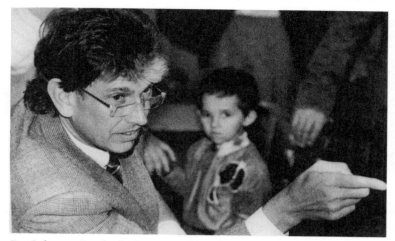

Dr. Salyer at Burdenko Institute in Moscow

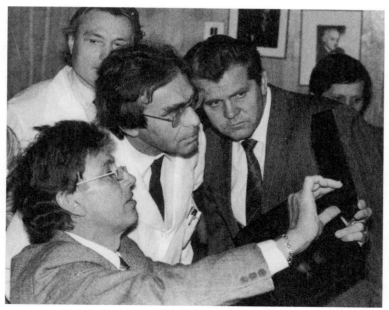

Dr. Salyer and Dr. Konovalov with colleagues

at the Burdenko Institute proved to be a remarkable one. We ultimately returned to Moscow five times over the succeeding years, bringing a team of surgeons, anesthesiologists, and nurses from Dallas, each time consulting, teaching, operating, and seeing patients from across Russia who came to us with highly complex disorders.

A group of twelve children and five surgeons also journeyed from Moscow to Dallas in 1990. The patients were children we believed could be treated best at our own institute—and that certainly proved to be the case—and we invited the Russian surgeons not only so they could observe the surgeries but also to acquaint them in some depth with the multidisciplinary approach to craniofacial and pediatric neurosurgery we had pioneered at Medical City.

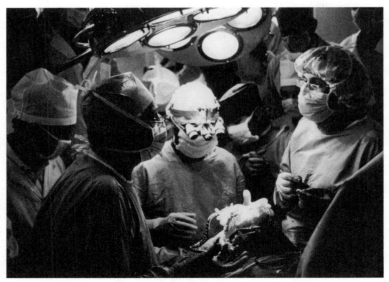

Surgery with Dr. Mutaz Habal in Moscow

I had worked very hard to create a center in Dallas that I believed was the best place in the world to care for children with tragic head and facial deformities and to staff it with people who were the best of the best in their fields. We all loved our work and were quite busy—and I worked virtually nonstop. It would have been easy for me to devote myself to my biggest goals—and to achieve them—without ever traveling out of North Texas. Yet I began to discover again, just as I had when I first went to Paris in 1972 at the invitation of Paul Tessier, that being out in the world was a wonderful thing. And as I traveled more, I quickly realized that the need for excellent reconstructive surgery was profound everywhere in the world. Only a tiny fraction of the children who required and *deserved* state-of-the-art craniofacial or cleft lip and palate surgery could travel to Dallas to receive it—even if money was no object. The solution to the dilemma seemed obvious, and it was one I wanted to be part of. Surgeons throughout the world needed to be trained in the innovative procedures that we had pioneered and made successful. And centers needed to be created in virtually every nation around the world.

On the heels of the success of what became known as the Russia Project, we took our first steps toward that end by reaching out rather close to home. Texas is an awfully big place, and patients from cities like El Paso or Brownsville had to travel six hundred miles or more to be evaluated or operated on in Dallas. So we began to go to them, holding semiannual clinics in cooperation with local plastic surgeons in Corpus Christi, El Paso, Midland-Odessa, San Antonio, and the Rio Grande Valley along the Mexican border. We held teaching conferences and conducted clinics staffed by many of our Dallas-based craniofacial team members at which we both evaluated patients and conducted surgeries. And we worked more broadly as well, educating local physicians and paramedical personnel about our work and making them aware of how much could be done nowadays to help the children with very difficult cases who were regularly brought to them.

Back in the days when I was working closely with Ira Korman and Humana executives to create the institute, one of the clear stipulations in our agreement was that we would accept charity patients, and each of us who comprised the core of the team was committed to this end. As the years progressed, one of the reasons we developed the busiest craniofacial and pediatric neurosurgery programs in the world was the fact that we could treat as many patients who had no means to pay as we did. All of us were prospering personally; the institute was making lots of money, and the financial folks at Humana were delighted with our accomplishments. We absorbed the cost of treating nonpaying cases without stressing the institute financially. It was compelling to me that so-called charity patients often presented the greatest medical and surgical challenges—and their treatments were therefore very expensive.

The more I traveled, the more I became aware of how fortunate we were to have the support of a company like Humana, and of how desperate the financial needs were of so many patients—in Texas alone and throughout the world. I continued to perform more than five hundred surgeries each year, but as I increasingly traveled to spread the gospel of giving every child a normal face with which to be seen and accepted, those needs began to stagger me, and I began to consider how best I could devote myself to ensuring that services were available for every needy child.

The Russia Project became a model—although that wasn't its purpose in the beginning—for a series of intensive and carefully planned outreach efforts. We mounted major projects in the ensuing years in Puerto Rico, Taiwan, and Romania, and I attended conferences and gave hundreds of lectures and invited professorships with the goal of spreading the knowledge base we had acquired in Dallas to everyone who would listen. And as Luci and I traveled—ultimately visiting seventy-five countries and every continent except Antarctica—another dream began to take shape, one I felt sure we could make real.

It's my nature to be optimistic. I'm confident in my talents and I don't take a backseat to anyone when it comes to resolve or dedication. I believe my dreams are essentially road maps toward what I can accomplish. And just as I was certain that I could find a way for thousands of children around the world to receive the excellent care they needed at little or no cost, I also was immediately sure when I met them that I could find a way to give new freedom—and therefore new lives—to Romanian twin sisters Anastasia and Tatiana Dogaru, who were conjoined at the head.

Claudia and Alin Dogaru were natives of Romania living in a small Italian city where Alin, a priest in the Byzantine Catholic Church, had been transferred. Their first daughter, Maria, had been born normally, but the couple struggled to have a second child. Claudia suffered two miscarriages before she became pregnant with the twins, but an ultrasound performed by an Italian doctor six weeks into her pregnancy was immediately worrying to everyone. The heads of the two fetuses appeared to overlap, and the doctor ultimately became concerned enough that he ordered an MRI, which confirmed his and the parents' fears.

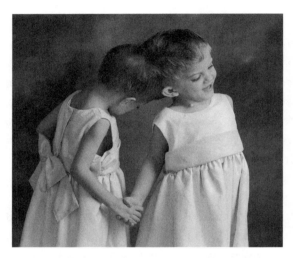

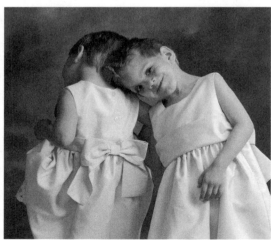

Conjoined Dogaru twins, Anastasia and Tatiana

Claudia was a nurse and understood how incredibly challenging it would be for the girls not only to survive to term but to live successfully with their skulls conjoined, but the faith she shared with her husband led the two of them to conclude that the girls were part of a divine plan—God intended something meaningful for their lives and the lives of those they touched.

Claudia spent the last weeks of her pregnancy in a hospital in Rome, and the girls were delivered by Caesarean section. "They were beautiful," Alin told me. "They were so delicate, so perfect, except that they were joined." Italian doctors soon discovered that being connected at the skull wasn't the girls' only problem. The daughter the Dogarus named Tatiana had a serious constriction in her aorta, limiting blood flow throughout her body. Her sister Anastasia did not have kidneys and depended instead on Tatiana for her renal function.

When the Dogarus consulted with Italian neurosurgeons about separating the girls, they were initially told little except that the possibility would be studied. After weeks of waiting for a decision regarding separation, Claudia and Alin ultimately were informed by the surgeons that, sadly, it would not be possible, and they were sent home from the extended-care facility where they were living and simply wished good luck. Claudia could do nothing more than resign herself to cherishing every remaining moment she had with her daughters, presuming that their lives could not endure very long. Later, as she related how we came to her attention, Claudia said, "But then I heard about you. Finally, there was a breath of hope—all was not lost. But how would we do it? How could we afford a trip to Dallas?

Would they let us take along our five-year-old daughter, Maria? There were so many questions."

When I first spoke by telephone with Claudia—after having examined photographs, CT scans, and other images—I told her I wasn't certain that the girls could be successfully separated, but that if the separation could be performed successfully I was sure we could find a way to meet its financial costs. I added that we were one of the few teams of surgeons in the world capable of such a procedure.

Only a few weeks later, Claudia and the twins arrived in Dallas. Alin and Maria had remained at home in Italy, and—suddenly in a very exotic place without her husband and attempting to manage the twins on her own—Claudia was understandably very anxious. But I was able to put her at ease.

"I was very nervous the first time I met Dr. Salyer," she later explained to a reporter. "I could not express myself in English. I could understand him, but he could not understand me. Yet he made me feel comfortable and I knew my babies were safe. He gave me a big hug—more like a father than a surgeon. And he had warmth in his eyes and his concern for my girls touched me very much."

It meant a great deal to me for Claudia to express such confidence, and I wished I could meet it with absolute assurance that the twins would return to Europe separated, healthy, and ready to lead rich lives. But as discussions commenced at the institute about the depth and complexity of their problem, some key members of my team began to express serious concerns about the risks.

The two girls' heads were attached almost at right angles, with the crown of Anastasia's skull extending into the rear of her sister's skull. When Tatiana was erect and looking forward, Anastasia was tilted sideways and her gaze was lateral. Although the girls had distinct brains, our neurosurgeons were quite concerned about whether the interwoven blood vessels that supplied them could be successfully pieced apart. And of course, the heart and kidney issues made survival after separation a vexing question as well. Yet in the end, and not without some intense discussions, I managed to convince the team to move forward with planning and research. I didn't want to give up unless I became utterly convinced that we would fail if we attempted the separation.

Certainly enormous risks were involved, including brain damage to either or both of the girls, the loss of one of the girls, or even the death of both. But Claudia and Alin—who, with Maria, was able to join the family in Dallas after a time—assured me that they were willing to live with the results, whatever they might be. They believed the fate of their girls was in God's hands, and they wanted us to try.

"I don't want lose them," Claudia explained. "But I can't just sit and wait to see what happens. If I don't do anything, I condemn them, and I could not bear that. They are so full of life, and I think they will always be happy. They are getting stronger every day and becoming unique little people."

During my long discussions with Claudia and Alin about the girls, it was fascinating to hear them describe how the girls interacted. They fought over toys and cried when they didn't get their way, just as all kids do. When one had a view of the single television in the apartment where they stayed, the other necessarily did not, for example, and one would sometimes try to push the other out of the way—without any possibility of success, of course. They jointly had discovered how to walk—and to fall—without hurting themselves or each other.

They struggled against their mutual confinement but nonetheless found ways to develop distinct personalities and senses of themselves as unique beings, each separate from the other. "Anastasia is bossy and pushes the two," Claudia explained, "and Tatiana usually goes along with her. Of course, Tatiana really has no other choice. Anastasia is facing out and feels more in command of her world." Because Tatiana faced the floor as a result of her angle of attachment to the back of Anastasia's head, she was often dragged by Anastasia when she walked.

But ironically, "Tatiana is the more difficult one to control," said her father. "Anastasia, who gets to face forward most of the time, will respond to a verbal command, such as 'No,' but Tatiana is far more stubborn, uncooperative, and slow to respond." Hidden behind her sister and at her mercy in terms of movement, Tatiana developed skills at avoiding discipline, sometimes taunting her parents and mercilessly testing their authority. "At first I thought it would be Anastasia, but now I think Tatiana is the one that will be a problem in the future," Claudia chuckled, reminding me that a parent's need to put some space between two willful sisters now and then obviously wasn't an option for them.

By the time those of us on the team had completed exhaustive diagnostics, consulted myriad studies, read about successful separation cases, and discussed the girls and their prospects for many, many hours, only one certainty emerged—Tatiana would need heart surgery to repair her aorta, regardless of whether the girls were ultimately separated. The operation was performed by our pediatric cardiac surgeons at Medical City Dallas, and although they did repair Tatiana's aorta, limited circulation during the surgery caused some postoperative weakness and paralysis in her legs. In response, she received lots of physical therapy, ultimately ameliorating the problem, but it also signaled just how risky each step of this unique and many-staged procedure would be if the girls were ever separated and able to look each other in the face for the first time in their lives.

Dr. Dale Swift, the senior neurosurgeon in the case, increasingly was concerned that the separation just couldn't be performed successfully. His foremost apprehension was that it would be exceedingly difficult to construct sufficient venous drainage to allow a return blood flow from each brain to each heart. But finally, he devised a tentative solution he believed had a high probability of working, and we began in earnest to plan for the separation surgery.

Our window of opportunity was brief. The older the girls grew, the greater the challenges. Studies conducted by Dr. Derek Bruce on hemispherectomies performed in severely epileptic children found that as much as half of a child's brain could be removed and the child could still function rather well. Based on those studies, and in consultation with Dr. Bruce and many others, we estimated that even up to age five, the girls could be successfully separated and survive relatively unscathed through brain regeneration and readjustment.

For the first time, all of us on the team brought real optimism to the case; we *could* do it, and the girls *could* live independently from each other. The risks were undeniable, but they were manageable risks and we were confident in our plan. It was time to take our separation blueprint to the administrators of Medical City Dallas to secure their approval for the surgery and their agreement to underwrite its cost. But the hospital—mindful of its own agenda, list of concerns, and responsibilities—met our proposal with a firm and unequivocal no.

The girls would not be separated in Dallas, and I was devastated when everything we had accomplished to date was simply halted by an administrative decision that could not be reconsidered. I had enjoyed remarkable support from Humana and the Medical City administrators till now—they had been wonderful to work with. But this was a wall I simply couldn't penetrate, I knew.

I'd grown very close to the twins and their parents, and we still believed in the dream of the girls being separated. But it was a dream we wouldn't—couldn't—realize in Dallas. And in real pain and anguish, all I could do was promise Claudia and Alin that I'd do everything I could to find a hospital and a team that could make our dream come true.

My initial journey outside the United States in 1972 had dramatically changed my life. Watching Paul Tessier work and becoming inspired by his unwavering passion and his commitment to teaching his craft to other surgeons set my professional life on a course from which I would never veer. And Dr. Tessier influenced me profoundly once again late in the 1980s as I took the next steps toward shaping the life I believed was my destiny. In addition to inviting reconstructive surgeons from around the world to Paris to observe his groundbreaking craniofacial surgeries, Tessier also traveled widely himself. I'd first met him in New York in 1971, of course; he had traveled to Dallas in 1974, and throughout his long life he visited cities throughout Europe, North America, and the rest of the world demonstrating his surgical skills and techniques, sharing his knowledge with fellow surgeons, and helping to give countless children new lives. Outreach was an aspect of his life as a surgeon that he considered a fundamental responsibility, and I modeled myself after him once again as I laid the groundwork for the creation of what would become the World Craniofacial Foundation, which we officially established in 1989.

My goal—and the dream I was sure I could realize—was to create a fully funded charitable organization dedicated solely to meeting the needs of the half million children born worldwide each year with severe head and facial abnormalities that relegate them to lives of struggle, isolation, and rejection. And with Tessier's example, I believed that the best way to meet that goal was to support the development and rigorous education of craniofacial surgeons around the globe and the creation of self-sustaining centers in every major country, dedicated to surgical excellence, comprehensive care, and, over time, an exponential increase in the number of children treated worldwide.

Throughout the years, surgeons from many states and nations had come to Dallas to observe and learn—initially from me and later from our entire institute team of pediatric neurosurgeons, anesthesiologists, orthodontists, speech pathologists, and others. For years I'd also published and lectured internationally—as had Tessier himself, as well as Ian Munro, Ian Jackson, Daniel Marchac, Linton Whitaker, Fernando Ortiz Monasterio, and other founders of the subspecialty—but now I wanted to do something more. I wanted to create a foundation whose impact could extend far beyond the hosting of visiting surgeons and the treatment of children from around the world at our center in Dallas. And abroad, I believed it was vital for the foundation to do more than support continuing medical education around the world and the "mission trips" that were common among American physicians and surgeons, during which patients received valuable treatment but little follow-up or comprehensive care.

As Luci, I, and many friends and advisors worked to get the foundation off the ground and out in the world doing its work, we developed a several-fold focus. The foundation would concentrate its efforts on helping to strengthen the few craniofacial centers already established in cities like Taipei and Mexico City, as well as on creating new centers wherever possible. Each center would bring an interdisciplinary approach to treatment and would dedicate itself to comprehensive care.

In support of the long-term viability of each center, the fledgling foundation also committed itself to the establishment of an annual visiting professorship, allowing an internationally renowned craniofacial surgeon to spend time at several WCF partner centers over the course of a year, demonstrating surgery, teaching, and mentoring craniofacial physicians and staff. In addition, the WCF would establish two yearlong fellowships for surgeons who had completed general surgery and two- or three-year plastic surgery residency programs and who were committed to developing a career in craniofacial surgery in their home countries or in international locations with an established need.

The foundation's third and equally important area of

emphasis became its patient care and family support programs that would attempt to meet the financial needs of as many as a thousand children each year for medical, surgical, travel, food and lodging, and ancillary expenses. We would focus our patient endeavors on children in life-threatening situations who required funding for emergency surgical care, and we vowed in the foundation's business plan as well as in our outreach documents that we would never turn needy children away.

It was an ambitious undertaking, and it would demand fund-raising initiatives with which I had very little experience. We had established the institute at an existing Humana hospital with funding that came solely from Humana's own deep pockets. But the foundation would need the support of many thousands of people each year making small and large donations and sustaining their giving over time. Each year we would need to raise two million dollars or more to pay for our direct services, and the foundation would need a small but dedicated administrative staff as well. I would be the "face" of the foundation—its founder and guiding force—and that was a role I was eager to assume. But just as with craniofacial surgery itself, I wouldn't be able to succeed as the foundation's chairman without the support of a dynamic and committed board of directors and staff.

In 1982, my good friend and plastic surgeon Dr. Bill Magee and his wife, Kathy, who lived in Norfolk, Virginia, had been very moved on a mission trip to the Philippines by the enormous need for cleft lip care in that country and had begun a foundation called Operation Smile. By now, Operation Smile's efforts had spread to several continents, and its model was the classic mission approach: volunteer surgeons and support personnel from the United States and other developed countries traveling to areas of need in the developing world and hosting weeklong clinics where as many as three hundred children would receive full medical evaluations and a hundred or so would be surgically treated.

Later, a separate New York City foundation called Smile Train would join the effort by focusing its work on providing free cleft-related training for local doctors and medical professionals in needy areas around the world, using technology such as surgery training software and the grading of operations via digital imaging to increase efficiency. The two models were different—and each foundation has contributed enormously toward the effort to give children with clefts normal lives. However, I was convinced as we took the work of the World Craniofacial Foundation from the planning stages into implementation that our approach was the best—particularly because our work focused on the entire spectrum of craniofacial abnormalities, many of which are enormously complicated to treat.

In many cases, like that of the Dogaru twins, for example, a weeklong mission trip, or even repeated mission trips, could never have taken on their enormously challenging problems. Neither could a remote effort to train local surgeons. The *only* way children like Anastasia and Tatiana could receive the comprehensive and long-term care they required would be by spending months or even years at a dedicated craniofacial surgery—as, in fact, these girls and their parents did in Dallas.

We were a very long way from our goal as we set out, but it seemed to me to be one worth striving to achieve. Imagine if Anastasia and Tatiana had been able to receive state-of-the-art care in Romania, or even in Italy, where their parents were living when they were born. Imagine if other children, suffering from disorders ranging from Crouzon's syndrome to malignant tumors of the face, from craniosynostosis to Goldenhar syndrome, could remain near home and still receive evaluations, diagnoses, and surgical treatment on a par with the best centers in the world. One out of every four hundred newborns around the world suffers a craniofacial or cleft abnormality—and I imagined normal and fully lived lives for them all.

I had envisioned the successful separation of Tatiana and Anastasia Dogaru. No, the truth of the matter was that I had considered it quite obsessively; I'd planned for it in the greatest detail; I'd argued about it and prayed about it for almost two years. But suddenly, its success or its failure was out of my hands, and I felt helpless—or nearly so. Yet I had given Claudia and Alin, the girls' parents, my word that I would find a center where the surgery could be performed—one where the team performing the surgery was of the highest quality, and a facility that would willingly bear the two-to-five-million-dollar cost of the surgery. And I knew exactly to whom I would first turn.

Dr. Arun Gosain was a terrific pediatric reconstructive plastic surgeon based at University Hospitals Rainbow Babies & Children's Hospital in Cleveland, a good friend who had joined our new foundation's medical advisory board. In close consultation with Dr. Alan Cohen, the hospital's chief pediatric neurosurgeon, and many others on staff at Rainbow, Arun and the team he amassed did numerous further studies, examined the ethical issues, and—as we had done in Dallas—agonized over what would be the right decision for the girls. Ultimately, the team—one that consulted me closely at every stage—opted to attempt the separation, planning a several-surgery approach; the hospital approved it, and the family moved to Cleveland, with the World Craniofacial Foundation continuing to support them.

I was delighted. I'd long believed that the girls could be successfully separated—and I certainly wanted them to be if they could emerge from the surgery healthy and independent. Yet even if all went well, by now we knew that Anastasia would need a kidney from a donor after separation or would have to live on a dialysis machine forever. Universally accepted medical ethics could not condone taking a kidney from a child, so Tatiana could not be a donor. But Alin was an excellent match and, not surprisingly, was eager to donate a kidney to his daughter after a successful separation.

After months of intensive preparation, the first surgery of the several-stage separation got under way. The girls were put to sleep and special monitoring lines were inserted, as well as a hemodialysis catheter for Anastasia that would provide her with some basic kidney function during the many-hours-long procedure.

Dr. Gosain began the surgery by carefully opening preplanned flaps in the girls' scalp. Then Dr. Cohen performed a craniotomy, cutting through the girls' shared skull and exposing the dura, the tough membrane that surrounds the brain. But there they encountered a problem.

The dura was taut and tough, not supple and relaxed, as they expected it to be. The girls' brains and the dura that covered it were swollen—dangerously so—something that could have been caused by the anesthesia, the mechanical ventilators that kept the girls alive, or abnormalities in the complex vascular system that supplied blood to the two brains. The team was uncertain about the specific cause, but a sudden and worrisome drop in Anastasia's blood pressure made them suspect that imbalanced pressure in the blood flowing to and from the brain was the likely cause of the swelling. But efforts to increase Anastasia's blood pressure by tilting her downward on the operating table designed specifically for the surgery were unsuccessful and her pressure remained unacceptably low.

After eleven grueling hours, with no lessening of the swelling, and with Anastasia's blood pressure still at unsafe levels, the surgeons knew they had no option except to replace the rectangle of bone they had removed from the girls' common skull and suture their scalp back into place.

A few weeks after the aborted surgery, and on the heels of an extensive array of new tests that determined that now both girls had developed heart defects, officials at Rainbow announced that no further separation surgery would be attempted.

Dr. Cohen publicly voiced his belief that it was the right call. Dr. Gosain shared with me via telephone his great disappointment, but he, too, believed the risks had grown too great. Dr. James Goodrich at Montefiore Medical Center in New York—with whom we had closely consulted since we had begun to plan for the separation in Dallas, and who had led the team that successfully separated conjoined Filipino boys a few years before—was adamant in his opinion that the Cleveland team deserved real credit for discontinuing its efforts. And finally I, too, had to surrender hope.

Dr. Goodrich now was certain that the staged approach he'd used to separate the Filipino boys would not work with the Dogaru twins, given their anatomical configuration, age, and other factors. And even if we collectively had solved the problem of blood circulation to the separated brains and created a watertight seal of the brain's outer lining, there were many other difficult issues—reconstruction of the skulls, creation of adequate tissue to cover the tops of the girls' heads, the kidney transplant, and numerous general health issues—that had simply grown insurmountable.

We had tried, but we had failed. Yet the failure was simply an inability to realize our dream. Every surgeon must know when he or she can do no more—or that surgeon shouldn't be entrusted with human lives. And we had not failed the girls. They had grown stronger and their overall health had improved since they'd first journeyed to the United States three years before. Tatiana had received a critical heart repair and was gaining weight, and neither girl required special medication.

Not long after the final decision was made, I heard from Claudia. The girls were doing well, she told me. They were happy; they were living their lives. Just a few days before, she said, the girls—who shared a great love of animals— had been able to make a special outing to Cleveland's Metroparks Zoo, the two precious children as close as they had always been.

Chapter Six

Petero

I knew very little about foundations when I created my own, except that they were entities that raised money for charitable purposes by encouraging tax-deductible giving. I was dramatically aware of the enormous need around the world for excellent medical care for children with craniofacial abnormalities and cleft lips and palates—I knew *where* the foundation's funds I hoped to raise would go, and I felt certain that thousands of people would give generously if they understood the need. The challenge was going to be finding ways for the World Craniofacial Foundation to reach large numbers of potential donors and to move them to act in support of the children.

I knew from experience that perhaps the simplest way to demonstrate how magical postsurgical transformation can be for a child is to compare before-and-after photographs. Almost always, postsurgical images present not only faces that have become far more normal than before but also a renewed spirit, an optimism, an eagerness to move forward with life that's reflected in twinkling eyes and broad smiles. With that in mind, I decided to reach out to a few renowned photographers to see if I could interest them in the range of work we were doing at the institute in Dallas and had begun to do abroad as well, and, most importantly, in the children and their renewed lives.

I'm an avid amateur photographer and have been for many years, and I'd long been a fan of the work of photojournalist Eddie Adams, whose photographs had been published by the Associated Press, *Time*, and *Parade* for many years. He was best known, to his great dismay, for a photograph he shot at the height of the Vietnam War, one that captured the precise moment when Brigadier General Nguyen Ngoc Loan fired a bullet at the head of a Vietcong prisoner who was standing an arm's length away from him on a Saigon street. Like the equally renowned Robert Capa photograph of a Spanish Republican militiaman collapsing in death in the midst of a battle in the Spanish Civil War, Adams's photograph dramatically illustrated the true horror of war. But Adams, I would learn, was a gentle and sensitive man who was far more interested in expressions of compassion than in war, more committed to living than to dying.

I was delighted when he quickly said yes to my request for a meeting during a trip to New York City that Luci and I were planning. A few days later, he received us warmly, and I was able to discuss in detail with him the nature of our work—and the great need for it. We talked about the huge challenges children with disfigured heads and faces have to meet and about how, in many cases, these children leave the hospital after just a single surgery and their lives are changed forever. He seemed fascinated—and moved—and by the end of our time together, he had promised to come to Dallas to observe our work firsthand and to see if something about the work and its rewards might lend itself to compelling photographs.

That rendezvous in New York marked the beginning of what became a true friendship, the two of us reuniting at least a dozen times over the decade before Adams tragically died of ALS, Lou Gehrig's disease, in 2004. Eddie was a fascinating, world-traveled guy who covered thirteen wars in his career and received more than five hundred photojournalism awards. Despite being seasoned by war—or perhaps because of it—he was a humanitarian at heart and also was committed to mentoring the next generation of photographers. He hosted an annual event he called Barnstorm at his farm near Jeffersonville in upstate New York, a weeklong workshop where renowned photojournalists worked intensively with promising young professionals and gifted students.

One year, Eddie invited me to attend and lecture the group on the work of the foundation. I jumped at the chance—not only to further spread the craniofacial gospel but also to spend time with many photographers whose work I'd long admired. During those days at Barnstorm, Eddie offered to come to Dallas and shoot video footage we could use in our fund-raising efforts and as a prelude to creating a feature-length documentary. While he was at the institute, he became captivated by a seven-year-old Mexican boy named José de Jesus Cabrera, who suffered from encephalocele, also known as cranium bifidum, a defect caused by failure of the neural tube to close completely during fetal development, which in José's case had created a wide and dramatic groove between his forehead and his nose.

José had come to Dallas for surgery with the help of the foundation and a Mexican clinic and orphanage called

Mano de Ayuda (Helping Hand). On the day before his surgery, Eddie took José for a walk, and as a light rain began to fall, José told him that God must be crying. "Why?" asked the broad-shouldered, ponytailed photographer who had seen so much misery in his time. "Because he knows I have my operation tomorrow," the boy responded.

Eddie did his best to assure José that all would go well the following day—and it did. José had a great result, in fact, and he was back home at Mano de Ayuda in Morelia, Michoacán, before long—with Eddie accompanying him to photograph his return. It wasn't long thereafter that, somewhat out of the blue, Eddie announced that he and writer Michael Ryan were planning an article on the institute and the foundation for *Parade*, the magazine supplement that's included in more than six hundred Sunday newspapers around the country and is read by more than *thirty-two million* people each week. "Get prepared," Eddie rather matter-of-factly added as he gave me the news. "Your life won't be the same after the article." And I smile as I remember what an astounding understatement Eddie's admonition proved to be.

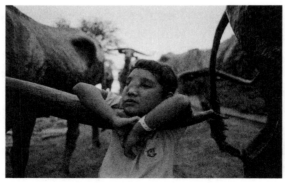

José de Jesus Cabrera before surgery

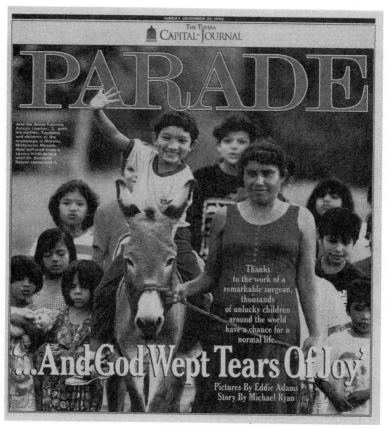

SUNDAY, DECEMBER 22, 1996

THE TOPEKA
CAPITAL-JOURNAL

PARADE

José De Jesus Cabrera Arroyo (center), 7, with his mother, Teodora, and children at the orphanage in Morelia, Michoacán, Mexico. José suffered from a severe birth defect until Dr. Kenneth Salyer corrected it.

Thanks to the work of a remarkable surgeon, thousands of unlucky children around the world have a chance for a normal life.

'...And God Wept Tears Of Joy'

Pictures By Eddie Adams
Story By Michael Ryan

Parade *magazine cover 1996*

I'm often convinced that the hand of God plays a vital role in the work we do. And surely it played a part in the good fortune that only a few weeks before Eddie's announcement, I had met a nationally renowned business development officer named Alexander "Sandy" Macnab, who was based in Chicago. When I casually mentioned to Sandy that an article on our work was forthcoming in *Parade*, he instantly understood the significance of that event and did a wonderful job of preparing us at the foundation for the onslaught of inquiries and donations that would result from such massive nationwide exposure. Sandy also initiated a database that would lay the groundwork for the foundation's fundraising efforts.

Then, early on Sunday, December 22, 1996—at the height of the Christmas season and at a time of year when people's hearts seem to be a bit more open than usual to the plights of others and the blessings that have come their way—there it was as I unfolded the bundled *Dallas Morning News*. I wasn't on the cover of *Parade*—it was *far* better than that. Instead, the Eddie Adams photograph that graced the cover of the magazine on that almost-Christmas morning was a wonderful color image of young Teodora Cabrera Arroyo leading a burro, with her triumphant son José sitting on its back looking great and smiling from ear to ear, waving his hand in enthusiastic greeting to the children who surrounded them. " . . . And God Wept Tears Of Joy," read the headline, with a tagline that added, "Thanks to the work of a remarkable surgeon, thousands of unlucky children around the world have a chance for a normal life."

You can imagine my delight—*our* delight. This attention was beyond our wildest dreams. Inside the magazine, Michael Ryan's article suggested that those raindrops in Dallas that day "must have been tears of joy. As these photographs show, José now has a face that will help him lead a normal life." The article also profiled a Cherokee girl from Oklahoma with Apert syndrome—which causes premature closing of the facial and cranial sutures and fusion of the fingers and toes—a Michigan boy with craniosynostosis on whom I was operating, and an infant from Texas with a cleft lip and palate; each of these children had very successful surgeries, and their futures now were bright.

"Salyer's goal," Ryan wrote, "is to perform a free operation for every paid procedure he does. Poor children now have to wait months for him to get the resources needed to operate on them—and Salyer worries that, with the growth of managed care, even children with insurance coverage will be denied the operations they need. 'It's getting harder and harder,' he says, 'but we haven't turned away any children yet.'"

Inside the magazine, too, were five more of Eddie's wonderful photographs, and I couldn't help feeling that Christmas had arrived three days early. The article concluded with the foundation's contact information, and of course, Eddie and Sandy Macnab had been correct. In the days and weeks that followed, we were *flooded* with requests for more information about the foundation, about how parents with disabled children could seek assistance, and many letters arrived simply containing donations. I was overwhelmed

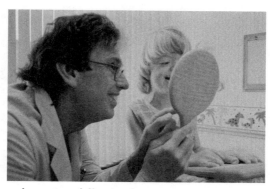

Dr. Salyer and a patient following her surgery

and deeply grateful, and suddenly it appeared that little stood in the way of the foundation's playing an enormous role in helping all of us achieve that goal of never turning away a child—regardless of where in the world he or she lived.

As it had for a number of years already, my life continued to be consumed by my demanding work in Dallas and my travels around the world on behalf of the foundation. My schedule was intense; it was exhausting, and I loved it. It was quite common for a trip to Asia or South America or Africa to lead to consultations with fellow surgeons about specific patients, and for those patients ultimately to travel to Dallas for surgery—just as the Dogaru sisters had and many dozens more.

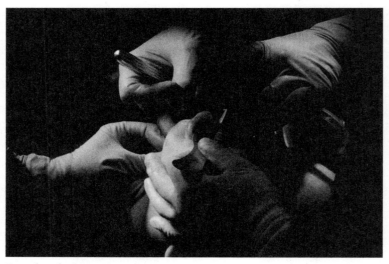

Four hands during surgery

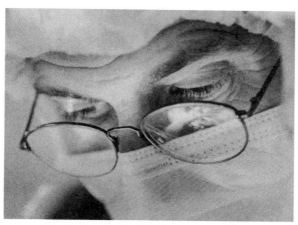

Closeup of Dr. Salyer during surgery

During a trip to Durban, South Africa, to deliver the keynote speech on craniofacial surgery to an international gathering of plastic surgeons, for example, I had met Dr. Andrew Hodges, a British plastic surgeon living in Africa who had dedicated his career to helping bring good medical care to the continent's poorest and most rural populations. He was eager to see if I believed a young Ugandan boy named Petero Byakatonda, who suffered from Crouzon's syndrome and was in danger of going blind, could be helped—and helped immediately.

Petero had been born in a remote village in southern Uganda. Crouzon's had caused his cranial sutures to fuse very early, giving him a severely deformed, steeple-shaped skull and forcing his eyes very far forward in their sockets, the eyes bulging so dangerously that the pressure was destroying his optic nerves.

From the time he was only a few months old, Petero's family had been searching for a way to help him. But because

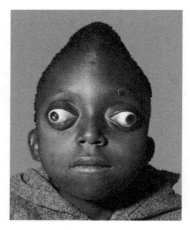

Petero, presurgery

the region's sole hospital was far from their village and they had no transportation, the boy had received no conventional medical care, and for the most part, his parents simply locked him away—not letting him out to play, create friendships, or interact with the rest of his family out of fear that he was somehow bewitched. On the few occasions when they did see him, other children in the village teased him brutally. And the teacher in the village's tiny school forbade him to attend.

When Petero's parents consulted a local shaman to see if he could break the curse they believed was the cause of his problem, the shaman sacrificed two hens and covered Petero's head with their blood—but the distortion of his head and face only worsened. A second healer in a neighboring village shrieked at first sight of Petero, calling him a "demon spirit" and imploring his parents to take him away.

Although disappointed, Petero's parents continued to try

to find help. Through a series of serendipitous contacts, the family finally heard of Dr. Andrew Hodges and his small clinic and took Petero to him. The British doctor understood the problem, but he didn't have the skills, facilities, or instruments to help. He had heard of me, however, and had read that I would be traveling to Durban—far from Uganda but at least in Africa—so he made plans to travel there as well.

I liked Dr. Hodges, and we instantly understood that we both possessed that *passion*—there really isn't another word for it—for never saying no to the possibility of helping a child in terrible need. Yet when I reviewed the photographs he showed me of Petero, I was dismayed. I don't think I'd ever seen a more severe case of Crouzon's syndrome in all my years of treating it. Andrew explained that Petero's vision had become quite compromised, and I now understood why. I knew, too, that Petero would need surgery just as soon as it could be arranged. I asked if it would be possible for the boy to travel to Dallas, explaining that the World Craniofacial Foundation could help meet the costs of his travel and his extended stay in Dallas.

Andrew felt sure Petero's parents could be persuaded to allow their son to make the trip. And they were eager for him to go, it turned out. But both his mother and his father felt ill equipped to accompany their son. They spoke only Luganda; neither knew a bit of English, and they found it hard to imagine negotiating airports, hotels, and the exotica of American culture. Andrew couldn't leave his hospital and his work, but he was fiercely committed to a positive outcome for Petero, and he began looking for chaperones. Several people came forward who were keen on the idea of going to America with Petero, but they wanted payment that seemed exorbitant.

Finally, a qualified volunteer appeared who could commit to six months in Texas to provide constant, nurturing care for Petero throughout his treatment and surgery—a young social worker named Immaculate who had just completed an employment contract at the hospital and who spoke both Luganda and English. She was looking for her next assignment—and a bit of adventure—and her genuine concern for Petero made her eager to join him.

Two months passed between the time in Durban when I first learned about Petero and his subsequent arrival in Dallas—precious time taken up with seeking approval from Medical City Dallas to donate services, arranging his travel and lodging, and many other details. And when he finally arrived and I met him for the first time, I was newly grateful for the opportunity to help this dramatically disfigured boy.

I'd never seen a patient whose skull was as pointed as Petero's—almost as if there were a dark cone sitting atop his head. His eyes bulged horribly, and a quick examination proved that he had effectively lost all vision in his right eye. His eye movements were uncoordinated, and because he lacked proper bony eye sockets, his eyes pushed out through his lids, exposing them to corneal damage from environmental elements in addition to the optic nerve atrophy he was experiencing from elevated intracranial pressure.

Ocular exposure such as Petero suffered normally requires early surgery. If he had received care as an infant in the United States, careful attention would have been given early on to protecting his eyes and releasing the increased pressure on his brain and optic nerves, and he might have retained good vision. In his case, however, without any medical treatment when he was very young, the web of sutures on Petero's skull and face had continued to prematurely fuse, leading to a whole series of ultimately life-threatening complications. When Petero had still been in Dr. Hodges's care in Uganda, he had undergone HIV, hepatitis B, and malaria tests, as well as a chest X-ray to check for tuberculosis. All were negative. But before we could operate on Petero, many more imaging and diagnostic steps needed to be taken. All the team members who would play a role in his treatment needed to see him and evaluate his condition, including members in general pediatrics, genetics, neurosurgery, and craniofacial surgery. Next, our neuroradiologist performed a whole array of imaging studies that led to the creation of a 3-D model—like the ones I'd created for Lindsey Gozdowski and many other patients—which allowed me to grasp in great detail the internal anatomy of Petero head's and to decide how best to alter it.

When treating children from developing countries, it's important to be sure they are in good overall nutritional health before surgery. Because he was accustomed to eating roots from the ground, Petero suffered from parasites that had to be eliminated before we could proceed. And it was also essential to carefully screen his hemoglobin level. Kids who are malnourished often have a negative nitrogen balance, which means they expel more nitrogen than they consume in their diet, causing their bodies to begin burning their own muscle mass—something that adversely affects wound healing. We did a complete diagnostic blood profile workup before surgery—and we would do one during and after surgery, too. And we typed and cross-matched Petero's blood and had three units of blood available for the first major procedure, as well as the one that would follow.

Throughout the process—and all the waiting—Petero was a joy to be around. He marveled at electric lights and elevators; he quickly began to learn a bit of English, and he and Immaculate soon developed a wonderful bond. She stood close by his gurney on the day he was wheeled into the operating room, and instead of showing signs of fear, the boy, who we believed was now about thirteen, began to sing a song in his native Luganda with a gentle, delicate voice. I whispered to Immaculate, asking her to translate the words, and she replied, "He is singing his favorite song. 'God, we

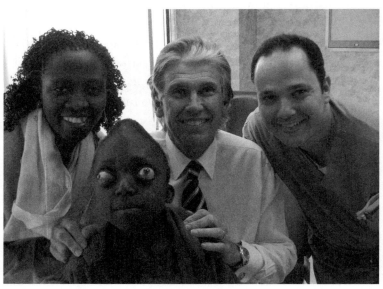

Petero, presurgery

have come in front of you. Please bless us and keep us. God, we have come in front of you. Please bless us and keep us.'"

Once we were finally inside the operating room, the first stage of Petero's surgery was to remove the front portion of his skull and reshape it, moving his forehead forward into a more normal position and positioning his brow ridge above his eyebrows in proper relationship to his eye sockets—a real key to facial balance and harmony and an essential preparation for the operation that would follow. At the same time, it was vital to increase the overall volume of his intracranial vault to allow more room for his brain and its lining and, in the process, release the intracranial pressure on his optic nerves that was threatening his remaining vision.

By significantly lowering the intracranial pressure, Petero's left eyesight could be saved—that was the good news. But the eye impairment he'd already suffered would almost certainly be permanent. Occasionally, patients who undergo such surgery do get a bit of improvement in vision, but in Petero's case, I strongly suspected that wouldn't happen. His right eye would remain blind, but we were all confident that his left eye would continue to give him enough vision that he could attend school and learn to read. His blind eye would remain in place and receive its proper blood supply like a functioning eye, and Dr. David Stager, our team ophthalmologist, later would do a bit of extraocular muscle surgery to allow Petero's eyes to move in a normally coordinated sequence so that they would no longer appear to be looking in different directions.

More than his vision and his freakish appearance was at stake for this boy, however. Dramatically increased intracranial pressure can also cause serious cognitive losses and, in extreme cases, death. Working in Petero's favor, however, was the fact that because he had never had surgery—unlike many Crouzon's patients his age whom I treat after earlier surgery has failed—we had no scar tissue to deal with, a real advantage. But exactly as in the cases of thousands of other patients on whom I'd performed major skull surgery, Petero did not possess all the bone we needed.

It's an absolute truth when it comes to entirely reshaping and rebuilding the cranium that surgeons never have enough bone—never. To compensate, we borrow bone from other parts of the patient's body and graft it into the position where it is needed. We take pieces of skull bone and split them in two, returning half to its original location and using the other piece as a single graft or cutting it into additional pieces. In Petero's case, I chose a third option, using a significant amount of demineralized bone—human cadaver bone—to fill in all the open spaces in his skull created by the remodeling. Demineralized bone has been freeze-dried and all its minerals have been extracted, leaving a porous matrix that nonetheless still contains an osteoinductive protein element that stimulates the body to regenerate bone within a framework. It's remarkable stuff, and it creates a scaffold, in effect. New, natural bone growth eventually replaces the demineralized bone, a process that normally takes about a year.

When we did Petero's first surgery, I didn't have an advanced understanding of how all the pieces of bone ultimately would fit together, so I had to rely on my own experience. A few things are basic in that regard. You try to use as many large pieces as possible—the larger the better. If you can reshape a big piece of bone, the task is far easier than taking five or six small pieces and fitting them together like the pieces in a jigsaw puzzle. In Petero's case, we had to work with multiple pieces of his own bone—plus the demineralized bone—and the situation was far from ideal.

The bone of Crouzon's patients is often thin and brittle, and reshaping a large piece can be tricky, requiring a delicate touch, particularly when the child is as old as Petero was. When patients—even Crouzon's patients—are infants, their bone is still supple enough that it can be curved or shaped as needed with a bone-bending tool. But Petero's bone was rigid enough that that wasn't an option. Instead, I had to make a multitude of little parallel cuts on the underside of the piece of forehead bone I had removed, making sure not to break it, working in exactly the way a carpenter creates a curve out of a rigid piece of wood.

A normal forehead isn't shaped in a perfect arc—foreheads actually have much more contouring than that—so nothing is formulaic, and there's something of an art involved in making the remodeling appear natural. You pare away four millimeters on one side, two millimeters on the other—making dozens of decisions as you work that can only be made in the moment.

The forehead shape I wanted to achieve in that instance was determined by the totality of Petero's face, by his ideal proportions, and by what I felt would be aesthetically attractive for him. Another surgeon might have made different choices, and each surgeon relies on his or her experience and skill set to get the best outcome. Even though I had a 3-D model to guide me, it was impossible to plan in advance precisely where each piece of bone should go. And because I was doing Petero's reconstruction in two stages, it was vital for me to visualize how constructing a framework in stage one would affect stage two, when I focused my attention on his face.

I wanted to give careful consideration as well to the structural differences in the faces of people who belonged to various African ethnic communities and the fact that different cultures and subcultures have distinct preferences with regard to proportion and ideals of facial beauty. John Kolar, our staff anthropologist, was able to help before the two surgeries by making more than 120 measurements of the angles and proportions of Petero's face and, using photographs, the faces of members of his family and his Ugandan tribe. With John's expertise buttressing my own, I felt confident that we were paying appropriate attention to what the facial standards in Petero's community were, and I worked diligently to achieve them.

With the completion of the second surgery—during which I performed a Le Fort III, rebuilding Petero's eye sockets, repositioning his eyes, and simultaneously moving his upper face and upper jaw forward—I was very pleased with the outcome. I'm good enough at what I do—and immodest enough about it—that I very seldom have a result that personally feels like a failure. Yet some outcomes are unquestionably better than others, and Petero's case was one of the best. His skull was now beautifully round; the sharp peak at its crown was gone. His forehead had been remodeled with his own cranial bone, and the back of his skull now was shaped by demineralized bone, which would be replaced by new bone growth rather quickly. His eyes no longer bulged, and they moved in unison; his face now was forward and fit his head; he had become a remarkably handsome boy. The plates and screws that held the new bone structures in place were made of polyglycolic acid and would completely dissolve in six months or so; he would need no follow-up surgery and very soon could go home.

Petero had adapted to his strange new life in America with enthusiasm, optimism, and bravery—and Immaculate certainly deserved a great deal of credit. For months, Immaculate had been Petero's constant companion, confidante, mentor, pal, and advocate. Articulate, charming, and spunky, Immaculate seemed to touch everyone she encountered, and her flawless onyx skin and radiant eyes also bespoke her special zest for life. She quickly had grown to love Petero as if he were her own son, and when she first saw him postsurgery—even with a complex metal halo to hold his newly formed head in place—she was almost giddy with joy.

She delighted, too, in the way Petero marveled at his

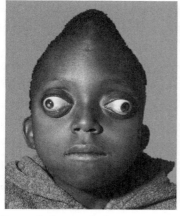
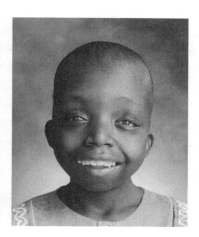

Petero before and after surgery

dramatic transformation. She told me about showing him photographs that had been taken soon after his second surgery. As he studied them, he pointed to a boy he didn't recognize and asked, "Who is that?" Immaculate responded, "It's *you*!" Petero looked perplexed, then took a closer look and shook his head, responding, "No, no."

"Look again. You'll see," Immaculate urged.

Petero's eyes widened as the realization that he was looking at photos of himself began to sink in. "I'm so different now," he whispered softly. "I've really, really changed."

After a brief final procedure to remove the halo and finetune the movement of his right eye, Petero and Immaculate returned to Africa, where they parted. Immaculate found a new position, and Petero went home to his family and his Ugandan village, where he would encounter those who had once shunned and tormented him. Although he looked forward to showing off his new appearance, we were aware in ways he probably was not that he would face a real readjustment to a life that lacked the comfortable modern conveniences of the United States he'd grown accustomed to—television, video games, cars, and three good meals every day. Both he and Immaculate would miss the warmth, kindness, and generosity of people they had come to know in Texas, and we would miss them as well.

Immaculate told me before they departed that she was certain that somehow Petero would always be part of her life. Perhaps they wouldn't see each other often, but they nonetheless would remain in each other's hearts. When I told her he was certainly blessed to have encountered her, she said, "I am blessed to have him; we are blessed to have each other."

I couldn't help giving thanks for the wonderful way my meeting with Eddie Adams and the subsequent *Parade* article had quite directly made Petero's good fortune possible. The foundation had grown exponentially in the years since the Christmas story about José de Jesus Cabrera. The foundation and my work had reached many millions of people. Without the funds that article had engendered, transforming Petero's head and face would have been impossible. The costs incurred in his case—travel, custodial care, food, lodging, evaluation, imaging, diagnostics, hospitalization, and surgeries—totaled $975,000 in in-kind and dollar expenditures. I was only one of many people who donated their services—American Airlines and Brussels Airlines donated Petero's and Immaculate's flights, for example—yet still, the net cost of his care was about half a million dollars, which, thank God, the foundation had the resources to pay.

A British film crew had been chronicling Petero's adventure for the Discovery Channel from the time of his arrival in Dallas, and his story appeared to be moving toward such a gratifying ending that it seemed to make sense for foundation director Sue Blackwood, Luci, and me to accept Petero's invitation to travel home with him for the celebration he and Immaculate assured us would await him. And what a wonderful experience it proved to be.

Sue, Luci, and I traveled separately so we could visit CURE International's hospitals for disabled children in Uganda before our scheduled rendezvous with Petero, Immaculate, and Petero's parents at the Entebbe airport in Uganda. Through interpreters, I met Petero's parents for the first time, and they were excited that the jet that carried their son would arrive in just an hour or so. "They have not seen photographs yet," the interpreter told me, "but they know he will look quite strong and beautiful." I instantly felt their warmth and gratitude and could tell they were wonderful people, and I was deeply touched by their appreciation for what strangers in a faraway land had done for their son.

The documentary crew was ready to film the reunion; Catholic nuns who had helped make arrangements for Petero's initial travel joined us as well, and the moment when Petero and Immaculate walked off the plane was one I'll never forget. His parents were thrilled to see him—their joy was palpable and none of us could keep from crying—yet he had changed *so much*, they repeated again and again. It was a miracle, it seemed.

The following morning, we stuffed ourselves into a Land Rover and drove for four hours to the Byakatonda family's very remote village. We were bounced and jostled mercilessly as our vehicle negotiated the rough, dry African terrain, but Petero didn't care. He could barely contain his excitement as we got closer and closer to home. Children ran out to greet us as we approached a tiny collection of grass huts, and Petero's four brothers and sisters stood ready to receive him—part of an officially assembled homecoming committee.

As the celebration commenced and Petero's mother knelt before me in praise and thanks, appropriate words escaped me—even in my own language. I was very humbled that I'd been able to make an important impact on the lives of these lovely people, so isolated from the basic amenities of Western civilization yet possessed with such joyful hearts. All I could do was smile and fold my arms around my chest as if to hug her, her family, and everyone assembled there.

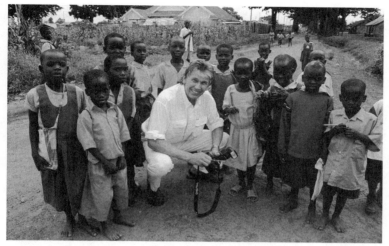

Dr. Salyer with a group of children in Petero's village

I was seated in the position of honor, with Petero to my right and his father to my left. A sunshade made of rough earth-colored cloth kept just a few of us from the glare of the hot sun. When it was time to eat, Petero was the first to be served, with a ritualistic pomp that seemed to make him very proud. He didn't speak—he was just a kid having great fun on a truly unique day—but his father did rise to offer his thanks to me before the village headman stood and made a long speech. Through the interpreter, I understood when it was time for me to stand as well. I told the crowd, "It is my great honor and pleasure to care for Petero, to cure him of the curse that had beset him, and to come here today to join all of you in celebrating his return. In every part of the world, we care deeply about our children, and that makes us all family, and I feel as if I was with my family today."

The headman then offered me two of the village's highest

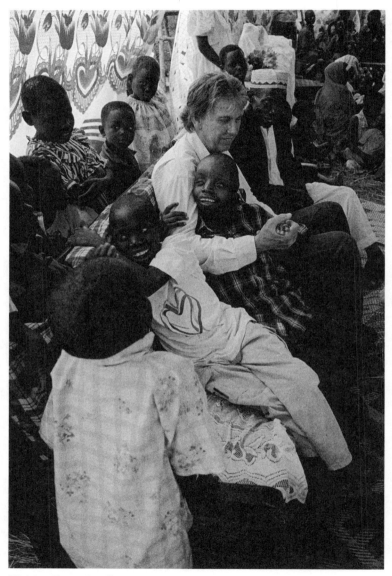

Visiting Petero's village

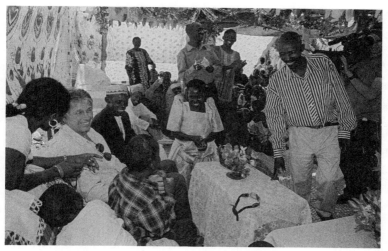

Petero's postsurgery celebration at home in Africa

honors—a live chicken and a lush, freshly cut stalk from a banana tree that was thick with fruit—so large I could barely lift it. It was a great honor to be given a chicken, I understood, and later I gave the gifts very discreetly to Immaculate's parents. They accepted the chicken and bananas gratefully, and I can honestly say that I'm not sure I've ever been more profoundly moved.

The wizened leader of the village of a hundred and fifty people addressed the group again, and his mannerisms reminded me a bit of a garrulous Western politician. He discussed at length his *own* talents and recent accomplishments on behalf of the tribe, then called for two other patients—one with a congenital abnormality and another with a tumor—to come forward to meet me, presuming perhaps that I could instantly heal them.

Mesmerized by the new Petero, the villagers personally

welcomed him as the formalities concluded. No longer a quiet, reclusive boy, he had evolved into an outgoing, gregarious adolescent who joyously danced at the party in his honor that followed. As drums beat out a seductive rhythm, he even managed to show off some moves he had picked up in Texas. And what a combination—the Texas two-step accompanied by African drums!

These tribal people had no running water, no sanitation, no heating or air conditioning, no electricity. Yet they seemed to possess a richness of spirit that was unparalleled, in my experience. And Petero himself seemed to burst with pride when at last he was able to show us his family's simple dirt-floored hut and the modest garden nearby where, before making his trek to the United States, he had planted vegetables, which his mother had nurtured. I was delighted that, at least for the moment, nothing about his time away seemed to alienate him from the compelling place that was his home.

The documentary team was able to record every aspect of that extraordinary day, and I'll always treasure having been a part of the poignant tribute to that courageous boy—one who beamed with confidence as he was accepted, embraced, and even revered, just months after having been feared, ostracized, and shunned. The opportunity to witness first-hand Petero's triumphant return—and the knowledge that thousands of other children have had similar experiences going home to other parts of the world, even when I haven't joined them—are the reasons I've dedicated my life to this incredibly important work. Who could ask for more out of life than to be able to help lift the veil of deformity and reveal such children's unique and shining spirits?

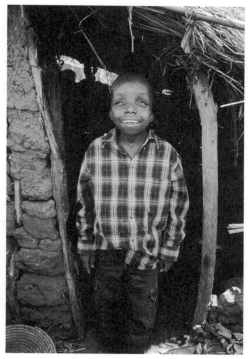

Petero at home after his surgery

I wished the late Eddie Adams could have joined us that day; I wished everyone on staff at the institute who had worked so diligently on Petero's behalf could have taken part in the celebration. But I knew they were there in spirit, and I was honored to represent them.

Like Petero, I, too, have been blessed.

Chapter Seven

A Normal Face to Love

It was 1986, and I was a reconstructive plastic surgeon eager to spread the word about the dramatic transformations we increasingly were able to achieve for our young patients, when the public relations committee of the American Society of Plastic and Reconstructive Surgery contacted me, asking if I would be willing to fly to Chicago for an interview on a talk show that was increasingly popular there and that had recently become syndicated nationally. The host was a dynamic woman in her early thirties named Oprah Winfrey.

The show's producers had shaped that day's hourlong show around the latest advances in reconstructive surgery, and I brought before-and-after photographs as well as videos of patients morphing from how they appeared before surgery to the way they looked postoperatively. Lynn Beaver, my early Crouzon's patient on whom Paul Tessier and I had operated in 1974, was one of the patients whose transformations I demonstrated, as were a number of other children with a range of syndromes who had had wonderful surgical results. Young Oprah Winfrey was full of energy and seemed fascinated by the opportunity for children to effectively start life anew, and before the hour was over she seemed to share my passion for the life-changing nature of my work.

Some years later, the show's producers invited me back, this time to join an hourlong panel with three people who suffered congenital deformity and trauma. One was a beautiful raven-haired young woman who had been born with claw hands, without fingers. She was articulate and engaging, and she and Oprah seemed to develop a quick rapport. The second panelist was a man suffering from severe neurofibromatosis, a genetically inherited disorder in which nerve tissue develops tumors, sometimes causing serious damage by compressing and blocking nerves and creating unsightly bumps under the skin, colored spots, and a range of skeletal problems. And I remember, in response to Oprah's question, it wasn't a pleasant task to confess that, so far at least, medicine could do little to help people who suffered from that disorder.

The third guest had been badly burned on his face, arms, and hands. With my background in burns from Parkland Hospital, my heart was quick to go out to him and to anyone who had had to suffer the extraordinary pain and disfigurement that burns can cause. Skin is one of the body's vital organs; it directly interacts with the environment and offers a first line of defense against external pathogens, insulating us, helping regulate our temperature, and aiding us in discerning the world through sensation, as well as producing vital vitamin D. Unfortunately, skin can also be one of the slowest and most complex of the body's organs to repair.

Each of the three patients on the show that day had suffered pain, disability, ridicule, and prejudice to varying degrees—and each of the three seemed very brave to me in speaking so openly about his or her trials. Although my role during the hour was rather small, I did get the opportunity to talk about surgical reconstruction—both in relation to their particular circumstances and with regard to a whole range of disorders that weren't represented that day.

Because I spent a good portion of the segment simply listening, I was able to watch Oprah in action, and I quickly realized that she was every bit as in charge of her show as a surgeon is in an operating room. I was accustomed to that authority—using it well is something every good surgeon must learn to do, even to love—but that day I was in Oprah's operating room, so to speak, and *she* determined the content, pace, and rhythm of our discussion. She was very good at what she did—and I was just one of millions of Americans who were beginning to understand that.

A year or so later, I was invited a third time for a segment of the show, this time focused on my patient Jacob Welker, who had had a severe bilateral cleft lip and palate; his premaxilla—the part of the upper jaw that bears the incisor teeth—jutted out in front of his palate, pushing his nose and upper lip into a grotesque and totally unacceptable deformity. A production team from the show had traveled to Dallas and filmed both Jacob and me, and I was able to describe on camera the two surgeries I had performed on him and what each entailed. With photographs, we were able to demonstrate how dramatically improved his appearance and function were after the surgeries, and I was delighted when he mentioned the help he had received from the World Craniofacial Foundation, which had made his surgeries possible.

Oprah hadn't quite become *Oprah* by that point, but she was well on her way, and I was certain that Jacob's mention of the foundation would immediately spur more of the interest and financial support that the *Parade* article had initiated—as well as the same outreach to the institute from parents hoping we could help *their* children overcome the challenges life had presented to them. And Oprah was not coy about doing a bit of cheerleading; she, too, lauded the foundation and its work, and by the end of the show she had made certain that her viewers knew how to reach us.

In the winter of 2001, Sue Blackwood at the foundation took a telephone call from a young man in Washington, DC, who explained that he was twenty years old and had been diagnosed with McCune-Albright syndrome as well as fibrous dysplasia, both extremely rare genetic disorders. Patients with McCune-Albright's often suffer from abnormal bone growth in the skull, abnormal heart rhythms, gigantism, hyperthyroidism, pituitary or thyroid tumors, and other disorders. Fibrous dysplasia is a bone disease that destroys normal bone and replaces it with fibrous bone tissue, often resulting in bone pain, bone lesions, and frequent fractures.

"I remember Shawn's voice being so slow, low, and distinctive," Sue recalls. "He told me he had seen Dr. Salyer on Oprah Winfrey's show back when he was in high school, and he knew from that moment he wanted to come to Dallas to see him, but he didn't have health insurance. Now, however, he had a job working for the US Treasury Department. He had health benefits and he was calling to inquire whether Dr. Salyer could help him."

Shawn Coleman had grown up in the nation's capital,

and throughout his life had dealt with entrenched poverty and racial discrimination, as well as the terrible stigma of suffering from two rare disorders that had turned him into a huge-headed giant. His father had left home about the time Shawn's skull began to grow large. Shawn continued to live with his mother, but a new stepfather didn't want him around, so he went to live with his grandparents, and his maternal grandfather became an important role model for the boy, loving and accepting Shawn despite his appearance. By the time Shawn graduated from high school, his skull had grown enormous—more than eight inches thick in places—and just as had happened with Petero, pressure on his optic nerves already had caused blindness in one eye and he was in danger of losing his sight completely.

At the close of that first phone call, Sue assured Shawn that the WCF would assist him with financial support that would make it possible for him to come to Dallas for evaluation and possibly surgery. Not long thereafter, Barbara White, a wonderful friend of the institute and the foundation, volunteered to meet him at the airport. Barbara and Sue—and all of us—were quickly struck by how gentle, calm, kind, and appreciative Shawn was, and he and Barbara eventually developed a close relationship.

He once confided to her that his sole goal in seeking treatment was to "look nice enough to find someone to love me, so I can get married." And I'm sure he must have said something similar to Sue. "More than his next breath," Sue told me a few minutes before I met him for the first time, "Shawn wants to look normal, just blend into the crowd—to simply be accepted and find someone to love him."

By now, we were seeing many patients at the institute

with rare diagnoses. When Shawn first reached out to us, I had seen more than thirty cases of fibrous dysplasia and would eventually treat about seventy more, but I'd never seen it in combination with McCune-Albright syndrome. As I would have expected, Shawn told me that he'd had lots of bone fractures during childhood, and on examination it was obvious that he also suffered severe scoliosis of his spine and thorax. I had never seen such a large head in my life; he looked at first sight like an ordinary twenty-year-old man, but one with a large, dark pumpkin atop his shoulders.

My heart ached for Shawn because I knew how shocked people he encountered must have been by his appearance, and I could only imagine how he was treated. Very unusual cases like Shawn's had always been of tremendous interest to me, most particularly an infamous young man in Victorian England whose life and medical history I had researched in some depth and about whom I had lectured over the years.

Joseph Merrick was born on August 5, 1862, in Leicester, England, and was completely normal until the age of three. But by the time he was twelve, when his mother died, he had deformities that had become severe. His skin had grown thick and lumpy; his lips, hands, feet, and head had grown grotesquely out of proportion, and a huge bony lump jutted out on his forehead. When his father remarried, his horrified stepmother expelled him from the house, and young Joseph began struggling not only against his terrible deformity but against homelessness and starvation as well.

Despite hiding his face behind a burlap mask, Merrick still had to endure the constant harassment of local children and adults, and he eventually ended up in the Leicester

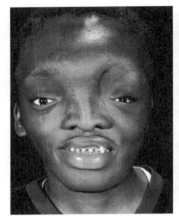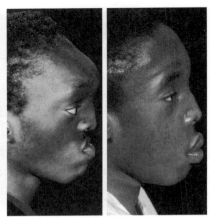

Shawn preoperation   *Shawn pre- and postoperation*

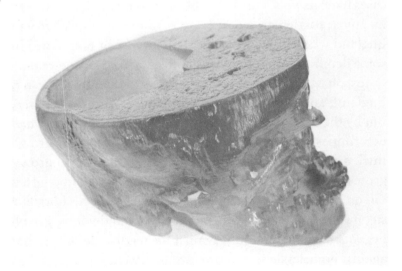

Model of Shawn's skull

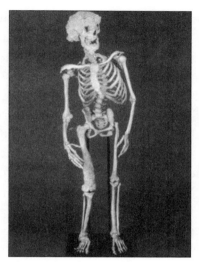

Joseph Merrick's skeleton

Union Workhouse. But because of his progressing deformity, he became physically unable to work, and he contacted an impresario named Sam Torr, proposing that Torr exhibit him. Torr agreed, and Merrick—a kind and gentle man by all accounts—became "the Elephant Man."

While on exhibit on Mile End Road in London a few years later, Merrick met Dr. Frederick Treves, but he wouldn't agree to be examined by the physician. Sometime later, police found Merrick at the Liverpool Street railway station, unable to speak because of a bronchial infection. But he did show the authorities the business card Dr. Treves had left with him. Treves arranged for Merrick to be given permanent quarters in the Royal London Hospital, where he was on staff, and Merrick was cared for there until his death at the age of twenty-seven—accidentally breaking his neck as he slept one night because of the massive weight of his head.

Although physicians and surgeons had speculated for many years that Merrick suffered from a disease called neurofibromatosis, Dr. Michael Cohen—a genetic syndromologist based at Dalhousie University in Halifax, Nova Scotia, with whom I had lectured in various parts of the world on several occasions—was the first to describe what he labeled Proteus syndrome in 1979. And he suspected that it, in fact, was the cause of Merrick's tragic life.

In 2003, Dr. Charis Eng, director of the Division of Human Genetics at Ohio State University, announced that DNA tests on samples of Merrick's hair and bone had proved that Merrick definitely suffered Proteus syndrome and that he may have had neurofibromatosis type 1 as well.

I know my fascination with Joseph Merrick played a role in the personal and emotional ways I was fascinated by Shawn. Something ineffable seemed to link him to Merrick; both young men possessed a gentle spirit, and both longed very much to be loved. I know I was drawn to Shawn, too, because he had always suffered from asthma, as I had as a boy. Much about this gentle giant who lived so alone in the world made me ache for him, even as I began to treat him and try to give him a better life.

I'd made what I thought was a realistic assessment of Shawn and his predicament during his first trip to Dallas. But it wasn't until a bit later—when, for the first time, I held a 3-D stereolithographic model of his skull in my hands— that I was truly struck by the enormous size of his head. It was *far* larger than any human skull I had ever seen, even in photographs. Even more arresting was my discovery that his brain resided entirely in the back of his head—in only a third of the space a brain normally occupies. The rest of the space that normally would have contained his brain was filled solely with his thickened skull, occupying the entire anterior and middle cranial fossa with more fibrous diseased bone than at first I could believe, fully eight inches thick in some areas.

As a four-year-old, Shawn had undergone an operation during which surgeons attempted to remove much of the fibrous bone that had grown in his skull, but the surgery was unsuccessful. It and a second surgery performed three years later had, in fact, made his situation worse by inhibiting the growth of his left eye socket and upper jaw while the dramatic overgrowth of his brow and the rest of his skull continued.

With fibrous dysplasia, a benign bony tumor often invades and displaces the eyes and compresses the optic nerves. Without treatment, the inevitable result is blindness, and that would be the certain outcome for Shawn unless we were able to help. Drs. Derek Bruce and Ken Shapiro, the institute's pediatric neurosurgeons, had demonstrated in more than twenty-five surgical cases by that time that optic nerves could be decompressed and vision saved via resection of the bony tumor surrounding them. But the procedure would be a daunting task in Shawn's case because both his optic nerves were surrounded by so *much* bone.

Before my colleagues' new developments at the institute,

the normal surgical approach to this problem would have been to reach the bone surrounding the optic nerve intracranially—by cutting a hole in the skull—but this method was difficult for most neurosurgeons and often was unsuccessful. Bruce and Shapiro, however, had found that by going in trans-orbitally, they could create a pathway that would allow them to cut away the bone that needed to be removed and decompress the optic nerve without disturbing the brain or the dura surrounding it—in general a much safer approach.

With Shawn, the stark complication was that his optic canal was embedded in *six inches* of enlarged cranial bone, and because his eyes were so dramatically swollen, trans-orbital access was almost impossible. Even with the best 3-D modeling, it would be virtually impossible to find our way through the bone to the right location, then "unroof" his optic nerve, removing the intense pressure the bone was placing on it and saving his vision.

So in February 2001, Dr. Shapiro and I opened Shawn's skull and began what we knew would be a challenging day of surgery, entering his head intracranially, reaching his right optic nerve, and decompressing it by removing the bone pressing against it. With that success, we forged on, also removing extensive portions of the massive bone of his skull, providing much more room for his brain, and removing the bone that caused his forehead to protrude severely, giving it a far more normal contour.

Although Shawn already had lost vision in his left eye, we also devoted our attention to his malformed left orbit and performed medial and lateral canthopexies on the eye itself, repositioning both eyes onto the same horizontal plane and squaring them on his face. It was a big day, but a very successful one, and I was delighted with how well everything had gone.

It's difficult to describe how gratifying it was to be present when Shawn first saw the results of our work. He was a young man of few words, but he was clearly overwhelmed, and he ultimately was pleased enough with the results that we began to talk about moving his jaws into a normal position as well.

Several months later, I performed a distraction surgery much like the one I'd done for Lindsey Gozdowski and hundreds of other patients, severing Shawn's upper jaw and anchoring a metal appliance to the separated bones that, little by little, would create a gap where new bone would grow. Over a number of weeks of distraction, we were able to move his upper jaw forward fully three centimeters—a substantial distance—and combined with some additional contouring of his facial skeleton, the results were every bit as dramatic as the first surgery. Shawn was elated—and we all were as well. He looked remarkably different than when we first had met him; he was joyous, and our collective spirits soared.

Shawn continued to work as a computer specialist at the Treasury Department and to attend college classes at night, a taxing schedule he endured with the grace and good nature that were his hallmark. He was determined to make a life for himself, and his prospects looked brighter now than they ever had before. But a particular tragedy of a disease like fibrous dysplasia is that the overgrowth of bone cannot be halted; it simply continues its mad replicating course, and new tumorous growth often returns with a cruel vengeance in areas where it has been removed.

We were all saddened when, only a year after his second surgery, Shawn called Sue Blackwood at the foundation with the news that the vision in his remaining eye was rapidly deteriorating. And yes, he admitted when I spoke with him soon thereafter, his forehead and the areas around his eyes had begun to grow much bigger again. "We both know what this means," I told him. "We're going to have to do another surgery much like the first one. It's going to be even more challenging this time. And we can't guarantee the outcome, Shawn. But we need to do it soon."

In 2003, Shawn flew back to Dallas and Barbara White met him at the airport, just as she had many times before. He was in good spirits—no one had ever seen him otherwise— but all of us, including Shawn, knew that saving his sight was not going to be easy. And in the operating room a couple of days later, Ken Shapiro, Raul Barceló, anesthesiologist Jim Rothschiller, and I were heartsick when we failed. In the midst of our heroic effort to remove the new bone that was compressing Shawn's optic nerve, the nerve itself had been crushed beyond repair. His sight was lost.

How long thereafter might Shawn have been able to see if we had opted *not* to operate again? Two months, five months, six, perhaps, before he was entirely blind. His rapidly deteriorating vision was stark evidence that the frenzied growth of bone would have utterly destroyed his optic nerve before long. But that truth didn't make us feel a bit better. Failure of any kind is always unacceptable. It happens, and thank God it happens rarely, but it's an outcome with which neither I nor my colleagues ever rest easily. We left the operating room that day feeling defeated and deeply sorry to have failed to help a young man who had greatly endeared himself to us, a young man who was huge and strong and endlessly gentle.

Sometime well after Shawn had returned to Washington—where, just as I might have predicted, he was able to retain his job and continue going to school as part of his remarkable adjustment to becoming blind—Barbara White shared with me a conversation she had had with him only hours after he learned that he would not see again.

"Mrs. White," he had told her. "I think I'm going to kill myself. This is too much. Now I don't have anything." But she boldly disagreed, telling Shawn that at least he still had his strength. "You're one of the strongest people I've ever known and you're going to find a way forward. I know you are. I *expect* you to, and I will help you in every way I can."

As they spoke, a nurse's assistant who didn't know her stopped at Shawn's bed and told Barbara that she would need to leave. Only family members were permitted in the intensive care unit, and because Shawn's skin was dark and Barbara's was light, the young woman presumed they were not related. But Barbara wasn't going anywhere. "Just treat me like I'm his mother," she told the assistant, who nodded and left them alone.

"Mrs. White, I wish you *were* my mother," Shawn told her a moment later, and Barbara said she had no other words except to simply repeat herself. "Just treat me like I am."

Houeyi Edah had never heard of Oprah Winfrey before initiating her long journey to Dallas; she had never seen

Oprah's television show, nor did she know what a television was. Eleven-year-old Houeyi lived in the remote outback in Benin, a tiny country in western Africa. Like Petero's family in distant Uganda, Houeyi and her parents and brothers and sisters lived without any modern conveniences and subsisted on roots, nuts, corn, and the few other vegetables they could grow, as well as the eggs and meat of chickens.

Houeyi had begun having unbearable headaches when she was five. Then her head and the left side of her face began to swell, and the swelling never abated. The headaches became more frequent and more debilitating, and as a huge tumor began eclipsing her daughter's face, Houeyi's mother, Beatrice, sought help from the only health practitioner in their remote village—the local shaman. As had happened in Petero's case, the shaman believed the ritual sacrifice of a chicken would rid the girl of the spirits that had invaded her. But nothing halted the rapid expansion of the tumor that now dramatically threatened the vision in Houeyi's left eye.

Then, at last, Houeyi's uncle heard that a Mercy Ship would soon be docking in Benin's port city of Cotonou, and doctors on board would consult and treat Beninese people who suffered a wide range of serious medical problems. In the summer of 2001, Houeyi and her mother walked twenty miles, then traveled by bus to reach Cotonou, where they waited in the blistering sun for days with more than three thousand others who hoped they would be admitted on board the ship *Anastasis* for medical screening and treatment. As they waited, the shy girl stood nervously and self-consciously, her head draped in bright yellow fabric to shroud her not just from the sun but from the ridicule of others. She had never grown comfortable with the taunting she received because of the grossly ballooning tumor that now distorted her forehead and dramatically displaced her left eye.

When it finally came Houeyi's turn to be examined, Dr. Gary Parker, one of the surgeons on the ship, was able to explain to her and her mother via a translator that she suffered from what he called a cyst, an abnormal growth that had formed inside her skull; unless treated, it would continue to expand and pose terrible risks to her. Houeyi likely would need a number of surgeries to remove the cyst and reconstruct her face so she could look normal again, he said. But the surgeries were too complex to be performed on the *Anastasis*; she would have to travel far away. "But how is that possible?" her mother wanted to know.

Dr. Parker explained that the organization that operated the ship raised funds to pay for its services, and other organizations around the world similarly offered medical help free of charge to people like Houeyi who needed them. He asked the two to return to the ship the following day; in the meantime, he would see what might be possible.

Mercy Ships is headquartered in tiny Garden Valley, Texas, about eighty miles east of Dallas, and people at its operations center were familiar with the World Craniofacial Foundation and our work. They contacted us about Houeyi; we felt sure we could help, and very quickly it appeared that Houeyi's vision and her life might, in fact, be saved. When Dr. Parker first gave Houeyi and her mother the news, Beatrice initially said she was afraid to go so far from home or to allow surgeons to cut her precious daughter's head open to remove the growth. But with a bit of time—and the more unacceptable the alternative to treatment seemed to her—her concerns turned to elation.

Many bureaucratic obstacles had to be overcome, however, before Houeyi, her mother, and a translator could travel. None of them had birth certificates—few people in Benin did—but without them it would be difficult to get passports or visas. But finally, with great persistence and the diligent assistance of the people at Mercy Ships, Houeyi was able to reach Dallas, where she would remain for about three months in circumstances dramatically different from home—where her family lived in a thatched-roof hut without running water or electricity and slept on mats on a pounded-earth floor.

Houeyi's yellow scarf was draped over her head as she always wore it when I met her, and she was reluctant to remove it to allow me to examine her. She was old enough now that she had grown deeply self-conscious about her appearance; I had to coax her to let me look at her. When at last I was able to make eye contact, the first thing I did was to ask her what she hoped we could do for her. Before

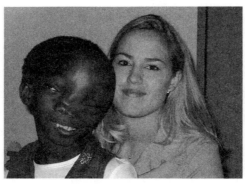

Houeyi presurgery with Kim Scott

Germain, her translator, could tell me what she might have said in her native Fon, Houeyi surprised me by plaintively replying herself in English, "I want pretty."

I smiled, touched her arm, and told her I believed she was pretty already, but that I felt confident I could remove the growth in her head, save the sight in her right eye, and make her look normal again—beautiful, even, as her mother and sisters were. She nodded but said nothing more, and I remember being very touched by her few words. Hers was such a simple and universal desire, yet her longing also bespoke deep pain, a profound and years-old ache that was not only physical but psychological and emotional as well.

When I began a thorough examination, I discovered to my immediate concern that the cyst in Houeyi's skull was actually a vascular tumor that was interlaced with her bone structure. Because the tumor had an extensive blood supply, removing it would be far more complicated than the team and I initially had imagined, and the surgery itself would be far more serious overall, necessitating numerous additional steps to ensure Houeyi's safety.

Dr. Ed Genecov, the member of our craniofacial team who was an expert in orthodontics, began the initial phase of presurgery treatment, removing eleven of Houeyi's teeth because of severe decay and associated gum infection. Because of the tumor, the risk of blood loss even in this simple procedure was significant. Next, Crys Sory, an interventional neuroradiologist, had to perform an embolism procedure, inserting a catheter into a vein in Houeyi's groin and moving it up into the vascular network in her brain, where he inserted plugs to cut off the tumor's blood supply.

A few days thereafter, we began the removal of the tumor

itself, and the moment Houeyi's head was open, the four of us who had scrubbed in knew that we were in for a challenging day. Although it was not cancerous, Houeyi's tumor had reached a very advanced stage and was enormous; she should have received medical treatment many years earlier. There was no guarantee that she would survive the surgery, given the magnitude of the tumor and its location, but we knew that without it she surely would die.

I had performed many thousands of surgeries by that point in my career, and there was little I hadn't seen. But I remember experiencing a rare astonishment that day at the size and shape of the enormous ossifying fibroma that consumed the small girl's skull. It was bizarre alien tissue, a sprawling, sinewy tangle of interlaced catacombs. We were daunted enough by its size and the degree to which it had invaded her face and the interior of her skull that we debated several procedural options for some time as we stood at the operating table.

A particular concern was what to do with the empty space that would remain once the tumor was excised. We ultimately opted to reduce the overall size of Houeyi's skull, but to leave the empty space to allow her brain—previously pushed back in her skull as Shawn Coleman's brain had been—to expand in the weeks and months after surgery.

Houeyi lost a lot of blood during the arduous fourteen-hour ordeal—blood loss we were prepared for but still had to work constantly to limit. But overall, we were delighted with what we accomplished and how she weathered the massively invasive procedure. When I looked in on Houeyi in the recovery room before she was awake, her face was swollen but symmetrical, and I knew her mother would be as pleased as I was with how normal she already looked. Someday before long, Houeyi, too, would believe she was pretty, I trusted.

Houeyi's healing was complicated in the subsequent months by a persistent infection that followed the initial surgery, forcing us to return to the operating room several more times to combat it. Houeyi also battled terrible swelling that took time to control, but otherwise she recovered well during the remainder of her five-month stay.

Besides the postoperative treatment, food, and lodging for Houeyi and her mother that the World Craniofacial Foundation provided, people throughout the Dallas metroplex supported her with their dollars and gifts. Channel 8 and the *Dallas Morning News* followed her case closely—she became something of a local celebrity—and well-wishers sent balloons, stuffed toys, and hundreds of cards. A Kenyan woman brought Tupperware containers of rice, palm oil, meat sauce, and *ugali*, a sort of cornmeal porridge, and promised to bring peppers from a Nigerian friend on a subsequent visit. Trainees at Southwest Airlines organized a car wash and raised $1,250 for Houeyi's family, an amount roughly equivalent to six years of income at home, and the manager of a Popeyes fried chicken franchise made sure she had an endless supply of the only things she ever really wanted to eat—their red beans and rice and spicy chicken legs.

Like so many foreign children who spent months in Dallas, Houeyi was speaking lots of English by the end of her

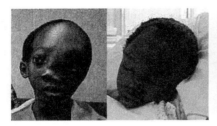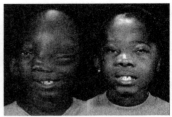

Houeyi before and after surgery

stay, and she wasn't eager to leave. She appreciated so many "people who like me so much"; she enjoyed many of the pleasures and amenities of American life, and most importantly, she liked the way she looked.

She *was* pretty, and she had abandoned the shawl that had shielded her face for so long. No longer afraid of being shunned or ridiculed, Houeyi now had a sense of being special in a very different way. As her wheelchair was being rolled into an exam room at the institute one day, I heard her whisper to her interpreter, Germain, and I asked him what she had said. Germain smiled broadly before he answered, and Houeyi—far from being the terribly shy girl she'd been five months earlier—smiled as well.

"She said, 'I feel like a queen. I sit in this chair and other people push me!'" Germain explained.

Unlike Shawn Coleman and Houeyi Edah, who began to lose vision when their heads started to grow abnormally in their childhoods, Jermaine Gardner was born without sight. Yet despite that disability, he was also born with extraordinary gifts. At birth, his mother, Jacqui Kess-Gardner, remembers, Jermaine

...had the most beautiful head of black curly hair I had ever seen. From the neck down he appeared perfect; however, his facial features were monstrous. He looked like an alien. One of his eyes never formed and was sealed shut. The other eye was extremely damaged and its white part was a milky mass of slime. The eye was about the size of a raisin and, because of the extensive damage to the eyelid, could not close. Jermaine's hairline was in a V shape over each place where an eye should have been, giving him an evil look. He had no eyelashes or eyebrows. His nose was disfigured, crooked, with nostrils that flared out and exposed their interior. His ears appeared to be unusually small and he was not at all active.

Doctors attending to the boy's birth gave Jacqui and her husband, Ollie Gardner, little hope that Jermaine would ever see anything at all. A Maryland ophthalmologist bluntly informed them, "Your baby is blind but has light perception in the good eye. He will need a cornea transplant, though it probably won't restore his sight. The left socket has no globe at all. I wouldn't get my hopes up if I were you because it doesn't look good and I don't think he'll ever see."

The Gardners lived in Baltimore, and at only five days old Jermaine had a corneal transplant surgery at Johns Hopkins Hospital, where surgeons also attempted to repair his eyelid so that it would close and protect his eye. The surgery went well, but within months, Jermaine's body began rejecting the new cornea, and during a second transplant operation the little boy's vital signs deteriorated badly and the surgery had to be halted. His parents were terribly discouraged, particularly when a plastic surgeon informed them that in addition to his blindness, Jermaine would need to wait until he was at least fifteen years old before he could undergo facial reconstruction surgery.

Yet the Gardners were fierce advocates for their son from his earliest days, and they devoted themselves to finding ways to help him reach his full potential. You can imagine their surprise—and their delight—when they discovered, quite by accident, that Jermaine, just nine months old, also possessed extraordinary talent.

> One warm and breezy spring evening, after [Jermaine's older brother] Jamaal had finished his piano lessons, I put Jermaine up to the piano in his high chair so he could "bang" on the keys. I then went downstairs to join Jamaal and Ollie, who were lying across the bed. Shortly after, we heard the piano and the song Jamaal had just finished playing. Ollie and I looked at each other and we looked at Jamaal. If he was on the bed with us, then who was playing the piano? We snuck back upstairs and saw my Jermaine playing the piano like he had been doing it all his life, *and* he was smiling. It was the first time he ever smiled.

It was a miracle—what else could it be called? How otherwise could a child so young have the hand coordination to properly strike keys he couldn't even see? How could Jermaine accurately repeat a melody he had heard only a single time? Jermaine's parents were astounded, and they were thrilled to think that music could become a way for Jermaine to connect with the world around him.

Before long, *all* Jermaine wanted to do was play the piano. As soon as he could walk, he would find his way to the piano the first thing every morning, hike himself onto its bench, and remain there all day, refusing to get off even to eat and falling asleep at the piano every night. His musical accomplishments seemed to grow with each new day; he could listen to a recording just once, then reproduce the piece almost perfectly. He fell in love with the music of Chopin, Mozart, Liszt, and other classicists, and could play their pieces beautifully.

As Jermaine's unique gifts became ever more apparent, Jacqui began to seek media attention for her son, hoping that shining a public spotlight on him would provide opportunities that would offset people's tendency to be repelled by his physical appearance. The coverage began modestly with a brief local television segment devoted to Jermaine and his remarkable skills, but then it exploded. The *Baltimore Sun* did a feature; *People* did a story, and *Jet* magazine did several. At three, Jermaine performed in New York on *Live with Regis & Kathie Lee*, and paparazzi even began to try to get shots of Jermaine at the piano from the bushes outside the Gardners' house.

When reporter Edie Magnus did a piece on Jermaine for ABC's *Good Morning America*, she became captivated by the young prodigy, and before long she was back in touch with a proposal. She had contacted the World Craniofacial Foundation and introduced us to Jermaine and his story, and the foundation had agreed to fly him and his parents to Dallas for an evaluation. If Jacqui and Ollie agreed, Magnus explained, the evaluation likely would lead to craniofacial surgery for Jermaine, performed by the team at the institute and paid for by the foundation, and the unfolding events would be covered extensively by Magnus and an ABC News crew.

The Gardners didn't need long to decide. They believed God had a plan for Jermaine, and although they couldn't know what its outcome would be, surely this outreach from ABC and the foundation was part of it, and they offered their thanks and their full support. But by the time I met Jermaine and his parents in Dallas, they had grown uneasy about whether exposing their son to the risks of surgery was the right decision. He didn't yet understand how different from other children he looked, after all; he wasn't distressed about his appearance. And would an attempt to give him a normal face risk his talent or even his life?

When the Gardners arrived with the film crew in tow, they met with fifteen different specialists, including a psychologist, a social worker, an anthropologist, a speech pathologist, neurosurgeons, and craniofacial surgeons, who would collectively assess whether Jermaine was a good candidate for surgery. Staff anthropologist John Kolar took photographs of Jermaine's skull and face from dozens of angles, making precise measurements of his nose, eyes, and forehead, and he underwent CT scans and other imaging procedures. When I finally met with Jermaine and his parents at the end of a very long day, I already had input from a number of others on the team, but my impression would matter most of all, and I was encouraged.

I explained to Jacqui and Ollie that Jermaine had what is known as facial clefting syndrome, and that unfortunately, they had received very bad advice when he was an infant. Instead of waiting until he was fifteen for skull and facial surgery, I believed that Jermaine, like the vast majority of young patients, would have had the best results if surgeries had begun while he was still quite young, allowing his growth to become an ally in the normalizing process. I explained to his parents that I could move Jermaine's eyes closer together, use bone from his skull to create a bridge for his nose, and use cartilage from his ear as his new nose's tip. I would move Jermaine's facial structure up and into a more normal position, would create eyebrows, and would consult closely with an ophthalmologist about whether Jermaine was a good candidate for prosthetic eyes.

Jermaine never stopped moving as his parents and I spoke. He was a little whirlwind, in fact, and his mother explained that he was only focused and quiet and truly happy when he was at the keyboard. The piano was his life—it was as simple as that—yet I understood his mother's particular concern that surgery could significantly risk his intellectual or musical abilities.

I tried to reassure her that a series of operations would continue for years, that they would be safe, and that over time, the institute team and I could make significant improvements in Jermaine's appearance. Our goals would be for him to be as physically self-assured as possible as he became a professional musician—a career path that seemed a virtual certainty. The more normal Jermaine appeared as he developed, the easier it would be for him to be accepted and to achieve his career aspirations. "And I'm the one who's going to protect the music center in Jermaine's brain," Derek Bruce, the institute's pediatric neurosurgeon, assured

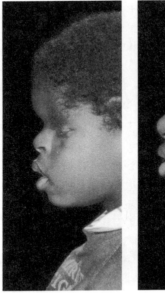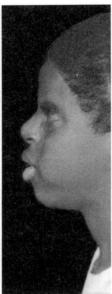

Jermaine before and after surgery

her as well in his Scottish accent. "That's my job, and he'll be fine."

It was business as usual in the institute's operating suites on the morning of Jermaine's first surgery, despite the fact that the ABC News crew's presence meant that many additional people were scurrying about in scrubs and masks. My focus was always obsessive, and it would have been impossible for me to be distracted—whether a single visiting surgeon was watching me work or whether millions would eventually watch on television. Yet I was pleased for Jermaine to have the attention, and for us to have it as well; the more people who knew of the institute and the foundation that supported so many of our patients, the more children like Jermaine we could serve.

Joining me at the table that morning were my scrub nurse Rosalyn Patterson—without whom I never worked—Dr. Bruce, and Craig Hall, a brilliant young plastic surgeon currently spending a fellowship year at the institute. Our plan was to perform a new procedure, one I had been contemplating for some time and for which I believed Jermaine was a perfect candidate. He lacked normal bony structure in the center of his face as well as its fundamental support for his orbits and nose. His misshapen forehead jutted out far too much, too, but I was confident that we could achieve a good result.

With Dr. Bruce taking charge of the initial entry, we removed the front of Jermaine's skull and remodeled it completely, giving him a nicely shaped and proportioned forehead. Once that was safely accomplished, I used the new technique I was calling a lamellar split to move the bony

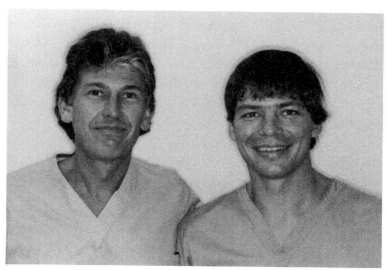

Dr. Salyer with craniofacial fellow Craig Hall

orbits of his eyes forward and closer together, using an oscillating saw to split the outer table of the bones of his face, allowing more secure and better-anchored reshaping and projection, and the creation of more normal bony orbits. The procedure went without a hitch—we were having a very good day—and we proceeded with bilateral medial canthopexies to bring the corners of the eyes closer together and improve their shape, with the goal of eventually fitting Jermaine with prosthetic eyes.

The operation and its many stages lasted about eight hours. The guys operating the cameras and boom microphones—who had committed themselves to filming the entire surgery—were exhausted; they couldn't imagine how we could work on our feet without breaks for that many hours several days each week. Yet they were still busy filming when Jacqui and Ollie finally saw their boy again and when, despite our assurances that the surgery had gone perfectly, Jermaine looked to his parents as if perhaps it had not. "Jermaine's entire head was wrapped in a bandage that was covered with blood," Jacqui later would write in a book titled *The Incredible Journey*, "and his face was triple its usual size. His eyes were swollen and he looked as if his face had been used as a punching bag."

But to both parents' great relief, within days Jermaine's swelling subsided. They could see the remarkable physical changes, and it became clear that Jermaine had retained his musical genius. He bounced back from the surgery just as we hoped he would, and he was *very* eager to get back to the piano.

Edie Magnus and the team from ABC were keen for him to play, too, and one midweek afternoon Medical City

Dallas became a mob scene. In addition to the ABC crew, who by now felt like colleagues of a kind, camera crews from three Dallas television stations were on hand in the atrium at the hospital's main entrance, where a grand piano had been positioned for the occasion. Reporters from national and regional newspapers were there—as was every hospital employee who could manage to slip away from work for a few minutes—and people stood elbow to elbow as Jermaine appeared with his mother to booming applause. The room quieted as he walked to the piano, then climbed onto its bench. His mother knelt on the floor in front of him, using her hands to operate the foot pedals the four-year-old couldn't reach, and for forty-five minutes Jermaine played a medley of Bach, Beethoven, and Chopin pieces that dazzled everyone present, including me.

It was an utterly new postsurgical event for me—and there were moments when it felt a bit too much like grand-standing for this surgeon's taste. But the benefits seemed to far outweigh the potential objections: the hospital administrators loved the publicity, Jacqui and Ollie clearly did, too, and Edie Magnus had a story reporters only dream they'll find. But most importantly, it seemed to me, was the fact that Jermaine was smiling blissfully throughout his performance simply because he was playing again. He was being his truest self—and that's something I wish for all my patients, whether the cameras are rolling or not.

Jacqui called from Baltimore soon after the family returned home to tell me that all was well, and that Jermaine was greeting virtually everyone he encountered with the blunt query, "How do you like my new nose?"

My answer back in Dallas was that I liked it very much. I was delighted with our results, in fact—pleased for Jermaine and his family and proud of what the team had accomplished. Much more remained to be done—but each of the subsequent procedures would simply refine the results of the initial major operation.

A year later, we did a secondary soft-tissue procedure to recontour and position elements of Jermaine's face, then followed up with more minor procedures over six subsequent years. At that point, I recommended waiting until Jermaine was fully grown to assess his situation and decide what, if anything, remained to be done.

Jacqui and Ollie agreed, at least for the time being, that surgeries to implant prosthetic eyes for Jermaine were not something they wanted to pursue—and their decision was something with which I was quite comfortable. Jermaine had worn dark sunglasses throughout his life—they were as much a part of his appearance as were the glasses that Ray Charles and Stevie Wonder wore, Jacqui explained. And Stevie Wonder had become something of a hero to Jermaine after he had been invited to travel to Los Angeles to perform at a surprise birthday party for the superstar musician.

By now, Jermaine had played for Nancy Reagan, Barbara Bush, and Cher as well, and he had recorded two albums, *Night Shift* and *Incredible Journey.* Jacqui had copies of both sent to me—and I liked them so much that I added them to my operating room playlist. In the years since, I've been mindful of the meaning of my work many times as I've listened to Jermaine's music in the midst of surgery, grateful for my role in his success and very cognizant, too, that the young patient in front of me on the table possessed unique and wonderful gifts as well.

I've been asked on a number of occasions if it really makes sense to spend precious resources of time, material, and many thousands of dollars to improve the appearance of someone who is blind, particularly given all the other medical and charitable needs in the world. It's a question that has always taken me a bit aback, in largest part because it ignores the fact that blind people "see" with their other senses, particularly their senses of touch, and because people without vision don't somehow surrender an aesthetic appreciation of the world around them or of themselves.

Patients like Shawn Coleman and Houeyi Edah were foremost aware of their abnormalities and their appearances

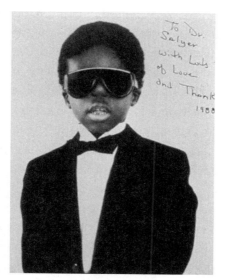

Jermaine in a post-surgical publicity photograph

because each of them once had had good vision. Both had a well-developed aesthetic visual sense, and to me it would have seemed cruel simply to somehow inform them as their vision deteriorated and vanished that the way they looked no longer mattered.

For someone like Jermaine, who had never seen with his eyes, the physical world and the contours of people's faces were things that he could profoundly appreciate nonetheless. Being blind didn't diminish Shawn's desire to have a face normal enough to be loved; nor did it seem fair to ask Jermaine to go through life with a dramatically malformed face simply because he could not see it.

Some people hold the perspective that the idea of physical beauty is, at best, a superficial one. Instead of transforming the faces of disabled children, they believe we should simply ask society to accept them. It's a noble ideal, but people are often cruel to those with disabilities. And I think it's a perception that belies massive evidence that cultural perceptions of beauty are far from shallow and instead are vital ways in which we give order to our world. Human beauty and expressions in its honor have been fundamental elements of virtually every culture throughout human history, and everyone who has ever lived has wanted to fall within a generally accepted range of "attractive" physical appearance.

When we help children who are otherwise "grotesque" look normal, we're doing work that's far from superficial. It may, in fact, be divine. I could tell that Oprah Winfrey inherently understood that truth as she focused her show's attention on children with facial malformations, and I wished that far more people did.

Patients like Shawn, Houeyi, and Jermaine remain so memorable to me because each of them radiated something special to the world, something anchored in their spirits that they were able to share with those around them. Yet that ineffable something wasn't created *by* their facial differences. It took shape and form because of how they met the challenges of their circumstances, and because their disabilities allowed them to understand what is precious in life in ways that many of the rest of us struggle to comprehend.

Shawn, Houeyi, Jermaine, and thousands of other young people have taught me an enormous amount over the years—about courage and self-worth, about dreams and their pursuit, about love and acceptance. What an honor it's been for me to thank them in return with my efforts to give them normal faces.

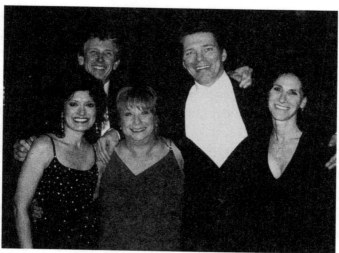

The Institute Celebration

Chapter Eight

Conjoined

It was an arresting photograph: two twin boys still less than a year old, conjoined at the crown of their skulls, positioned in a way that would forever prohibit them from sitting, standing, or walking. In late 2001, pediatric surgeon Mamdouh Aboul-Hassan, who had recently spent six months with us in Dallas studying cleft lip and palate surgery, sent an urgent email message with a photograph attached describing the twin boys he recently had met in a Cairo hospital. Dr. Aboul-Hassan feared that the brothers almost certainly shared too many brain structures to make separation even thinkable, but he wanted to be sure and believed my colleagues and I were the best people in the world to make that call.

I was immediately intrigued, but we would need *much* more information before we could even begin to discuss the possibilities of surgery. Dr. Aboul-Hassan sent numerous CT scans performed at the Cairo hospital, but they concealed key details. We could determine that the boys possessed two brains, but their brains were also fused in ways that were very worrisome; would it be possible to tease their two motor cortices apart in an immensely complicated separation surgery?

Critical blood vessels were phantoms—we simply couldn't see them. What we could view was a very large and utterly unique sinus that encircled the region where their brains met, one that appeared to have replaced the normal sagittal sinus that runs between the two hemispheres of the brain and channels blood back to the heart. How could we surgically dissect this strange circular pool of blood and remold it into two sagittal sinuses? Separation of the two boys would be monumental, but only a first step. Later, we would have to create skulls for each of them—perhaps an even more daunting undertaking. Eventual success appeared all but impossible, but I wanted to take a closer look before I offered my regrets.

When I saw my first set of so-called craniopagus twins on my first trip to Moscow, I was stunned to consider that two human beings with wonderful, very separate little souls could share parts of their skulls. I was fascinated—and something about the likely shape their young lives would take without surgery truly haunted me. Russian surgeons ultimately separated the twin Lithuanian girls, named Vehlia and Vidalia, and they lived, but it was vital for them to come to Dallas, where we treated them for a year and eventually were successful in reconstructing their skulls. Vehlia had suffered neurological damage during the Moscow operation, but she improved dramatically over time, and both girls have continued to thrive.

But the history of efforts to separate twins joined at the head has been one of very limited success. As my colleagues

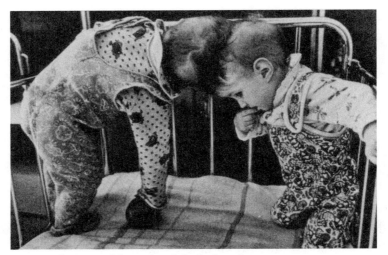

Conjoined twins Vehlia and Vidalia before their surgery

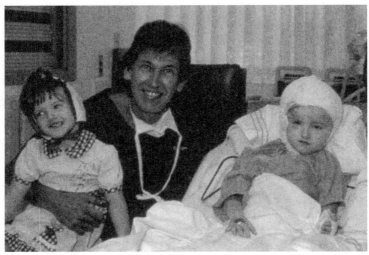

Dr. Salyer with conjoined twins Vehlia and Vidalia following their surgery

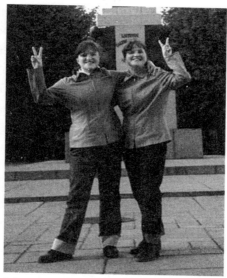

Vehlia and Vidalia as young adults

and I had discovered with the Dogaru girls, in most cases conjoined twins simply share too many vital organs to make separation possible, and when brains are shared—or even pressed tightly against each other—the risks become enormous. In more than thirty attempts around the world since 1928, just seven of sixty craniopagus twins survived attempted surgery without at least minimal brain damage. Thirty died, seventeen suffered neurological deficits of varying degrees of severity, and the fates of the remaining six are unknown.

Conjoined twins are always identical, developing from a single egg that splits into two separate embryos shortly after being fertilized. But the biological mechanism that subsequently results in conjoining still isn't known. Researchers once believed, logically enough, that the single egg fails to split all the way. But now it appears more likely that the egg does split completely and that the two embryos later partially fuse as their rapidly developing tissues intermingle.

Conjoined twins appear only about once in every two hundred thousand pregnancies, and most are either aborted or stillborn. Twins joined at the head are *extremely* rare, occurring in only about one pregnancy out of every two million, and for reasons that are entirely unknown, conjoined twins tend to be girls.

As boys sharing the crowns of their skulls, Mohamed and Ahmed Ibrahim, the Egyptian twins who were about to enter my life in a profound way, were probably the rarest babies on earth.

Ibrahim Ibrahim and his wife, Sabah, lived in a village where he drove a taxi near the city of Koos, five hundred miles south of Cairo in Egypt's Nile Valley. They had two children in quick succession, didn't plan to have more, and it was a surprise in the fall of 2000 when Sabah discovered she was expecting. At first, her pregnancy seemed entirely normal, except that her belly grew enormous. At the beginning of her third trimester, a local physician performed an ultrasound and then delivered shocking news: it appeared that Sabah's baby had one head and two bodies.

Horrified family members and consulting physicians recommended immediate surgery to terminate the child's life, but the couple couldn't be persuaded. On June 2, 2001, Ibrahim stood outside a delivery room, waiting as the infant was delivered by Caesarean section. Suddenly, he heard a cry, and he presumed all was well. Then he heard a second little voice, its pitch audibly different from the first. And he thought he understood: this wasn't one child with two bodies; he was the father of *two* new babies.

Ibrahim was awestruck when he saw them—his sons' faces were beautiful, but they were bizarrely joined at the top of their heads—and he was amazed that they cried at different times; they *were* two distinct babies. Sabah, still under anesthetic, didn't meet her sons until three days later, when she visited them at Cairo University's Abo El Reesh Hospital, where they had been transferred. When at last she did see them, she wept joyfully. These two precious babies weren't freaks at all; they were her sons, and Allah had blessed her, she knew.

The two boys soon became hospital celebrities, and virtually no one who encountered them could resist their separate charms. They continued to be showered with affection by their constantly attentive caregivers when their parents were forced to return home to work and care for their two other children. Yet their parents knew that if the boys were ever to be separated, they likely would have to travel much farther than Cairo and remain abroad for a long time.

When word reached the boys' parents in January that we

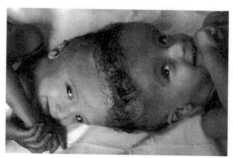

Conjoined Egyptian twins Ahmed and Mohamed preoperation

had made initial arrangements for them to come to Dallas, where they would be cared for by the same two Egyptian nurses with whom they had bonded in the Cairo hospital, the couple consented. They had never heard of Dallas, Texas, and they knew nothing of me. But America was a place where miracles sometimes took place, they believed, and so with both fear and hope, they bid their twin boys good-bye.

From the outset, it was clear that we would *need* something of a miracle if we were to succeed. I knew a separation surgery could permanently injure one or both boys' brains, but that children their age can also rebound quite dramatically from neurological onslaughts. But the clock was ticking. Before long, Ahmed's and Mohamed's brains would outgrow their ability to easily create new neural pathways and subsequently reacquire any brain functions they might lose. We would have to act quickly—if we acted at all.

With the constant coordinating efforts of the World Craniofacial Foundation's director, Sue Blackwood, we began to make the arrangements that would bring the boys to Dallas. We didn't want them to live in a hospital as they had in Cairo; they and their two nurses—wonderful, indispensable young women named Wafaa Ibrahim and Naglaa Mahmoud—would live in an apartment near Medical City Dallas Hospital. Medical specialists of virtually every kind would have to be recruited to offer their services without pay, and the hospital would have to agree to forgo hundreds of thousands of dollars in direct costs. Nothing was certain—except that we would see where the boys' destinies would lead them.

It's hard to judge whether the boys' flight to America was covered with more enthusiasm by the media in Cairo or in Dallas, but there's no doubt that they had become virtual rock stars by the time they arrived at DFW on June 22, 2002. Ahmed and Mohamed raised their forearms to their eyes simultaneously as paramedics wheeled their gurney from their plane toward a waiting ambulance—blinded not by flashing cameras but by the midday sun. Being outdoors, anywhere, was as foreign to them as Texas.

Two days after their arrival, the boys—great little patients, having known nothing but constant medical attention till then—slept inside the belly of a big CT scanner at Medical City, and we got our first images of the boys' skulls and brains. Their arteries didn't concern us, but just as we had seen on the scans sent from Cairo, their veins were a wild spider's web that interlaced both brains, something none of us had ever seen. Blood coursed out of one boy and into his brother—with vessels so entwined that we couldn't tell which vein would need to go to which boy. If we were to separate the boys, we were going to have to overcome by far the biggest technological and surgical challenges any of us had ever faced.

I was discouraged enough that day that my initial conclusion was that we should not operate, but neither should we utterly close the door on that possibility. Instead, I wanted to wait until we could develop technology that would offer them a better prognosis. But waiting indefinitely wasn't an option, either. I ordered 3-D models of the boys' heads, brains, and intricate system of veins—the same kinds of models that had become indispensable to our work—and I spent hundreds of hours turning those models in my hands, trying to determine a way to safely proceed.

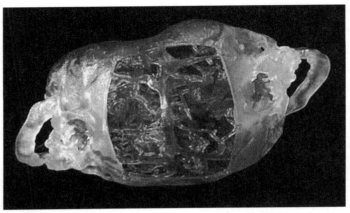

Surgical model of the boys' conjoined skulls preoperation

As I studied the models late into the night throughout the summer and consulted with local physicians and others in allied fields whose opinions were vitally important, I began to grow more optimistic. I spoke at length with each of the four craniofacial surgeons who had been such steadfast friends and colleagues for thirty years, and with virtually every surgeon on the planet who had separated craniopagus twins, peppering them with questions and listening carefully to their cautions and recommendations.

One of our important early tasks was to improve the boys' mobility and overall physical condition. Since birth, they had been forced to lie on their backs; they could not roll over or move themselves to a different location, and their immobility had caused distortion and flattening of their heads. To attempt to help—whether we ultimately separated them or not—we provided a multidisciplinary team of specialists who offered the boys a wide range of therapeutic modalities, including integrative medicine with craniosacral therapy, physical and occupational therapy, massage—and as much tender loving care and encouragement as possible. This program would continue throughout the entire time the boys stayed in Dallas and provided a remarkably valuable alternative dimension of support and care, one that worked in perfect complement to the more conventional therapies we offered them.

I was particularly encouraged in early August when surgeons at UCLA's Mattel Children's Hospital successfully separated year-old Guatemalan twins María de Jesús and María Teresa Quiej Alvarez, then was terribly disheartened to get the news that one of the girls had suffered meningitis and that now she could neither hear nor speak.

By now the boys had settled into their new American lives, as had Wafaa and Naglaa, who had become their surrogate parents as well as constant companions. Both children

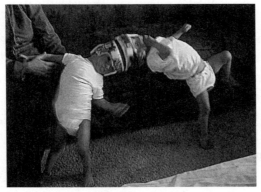

Conjoined Egyptian twins Ahmed and Mohamed preoperation at their apartment in Dallas

gained strength and grew healthier, becoming *boys* in every way. Because of the therapy they were receiving, they began to move and explore and discovered how to navigate their apartment, first spinning in complex circles that demanded amazing mutual cooperation, then scooting and rolling wherever they wanted to go. They sometimes would find themselves on their hands and knees, ready to experiment with crawling, but each time one tried to move forward the other was in the way, and when one tried to crawl backward, he was stuck as well.

Inevitably, the two learned the art of negotiation. When they disagreed on an activity or a destination, Ahmed, the bigger of the two, usually won. But Mohamed was loud and persuasive and could be counted on to protest. Neither could see the other, but they were, well, *inseparable*, and most of the time they were remarkably happy. And they had no idea that in a hospital a few miles away a group of us was trying to reach the biggest single decision of our professional lives.

As we increasingly understood how the boys fit together, Ken Shapiro, the case's lead neurosurgeon, and I became convinced the twins could be taken apart, although the endeavor would bring all of us to the limits of our training, our talent, and our good fortune. As we got to know the boys and their anatomies, the risks the procedure entailed loomed ever larger. But so did the images in my mind of what doing nothing would mean. My heart ached when I pictured the lives they would live if the crowns of their skulls remained connected.

Some medical ethicists argue that separating healthy conjoined twins can't always be presumed to be the right thing to do. Just like children with congenital blindness or who are born with absent arms, conjoined twins simply face physical obstacles others do not, those ethicists observe. Yet I had spent my whole career working to *remove* obstacles from the lives of my young patients, and this case was no different in that regard. The boys' heads were flattened from a lifetime of always lying on their backs; they lagged far behind their age group in reaching important developmental milestones, and it seemed impossible that they could always live in relative synchronicity, as they did now.

In long meetings with medical ethics committees, I repeatedly voiced my clear understanding that the separation could fail. The boys could die, or emerge from surgery with brain damage that could leave one or both of them paralyzed. Yet I also believed that despite the risks, each boy had an excellent chance to survive and thrive. I trusted myself and the totality of what I could bring to the several surgeries the boys would require; I trusted my medical team implicitly, and if the boys' parents wanted to move forward, so did I.

In making certain that surgery remained their parents' desire, we agreed that Ibrahim, Sabah, or both should come to Dallas to discuss the dangers and the opportunities for success with us in person. And yes, Ibrahim assured us soon after his arrival in America and spending some time with the sons who had grown so big, he and his wife still wanted their children separated. He was haunted by visions of his boys as men, he explained. "How will they get around when two nurses or one father can no longer carry them?" he asked. "How will they react to strangers' stares and looks of pity? How will they work? How will they survive?"

We were offering his sons the opportunity to live normal lives, he told us as he quietly wept, to marry one day and have children of their own, and Ibrahim couldn't deny them that possibility, he said.

Ibrahim was a bit puzzled when his authorization didn't immediately lead to surgery. But in the spring of 2003, just as each of his sons was rather miraculously taking his first step while his father or one of the nurses held the other one aloft, much remained to be determined.

The team of pediatric neurosurgeons headed by Ken Shapiro wanted to perform the separation at Children's Medical Center in Dallas, which had equipment—including a device that would act like a satellite positioning system, demonstrating for them the pinpoint locations of tiny blood vessels—that Medical City Dallas didn't have. But administrators at Children's wanted to consider whether it was fair to indigent American patients who couldn't afford care if the hospital donated two million dollars or more in surgical and postoperative care to two little boys from Egypt. The hospital's budget, like those of health institutions everywhere, was already stretched to the breaking point.

Yet how could a pediatric hospital *ever* justify turning away such uniquely needy children? For four months, I endured what seemed like an endless series of meetings— something I often find far more challenging than surgery— and then, at last, the executives at Children's made their decision: the surgery could take place at the hospital, but it would charge one hundred twenty-five thousand dollars to cover its most basic costs. Ibrahim was stunned. Where would he find that kind of money? The World Craniofacial Foundation didn't have that much available cash, and even if it did, our guidelines would have prohibited direct payment for individual patients' medical care. Just two years after the attacks of September 11, 2001, it wasn't clear either whether a broad appeal asking the general public to assist two Muslim children would succeed. Yet at a quickly organized fund-raiser at the Dallas Central Mosque in April, Ibrahim wept again when the people who were present, plus hundreds more across Texas, pledged nearly three hundred twenty-five thousand dollars to enable the surgery to move forward and give his sons the opportunity to live separate lives.

At last surgery was scheduled—ten months after the boys had arrived from Egypt—but *this* operation, one that would be performed at Medical City Dallas, would be routine in comparison with the separation and skull construction surgeries that would follow. Before we could separate the twins, each needed skin that would cover his brain and the new skull sections we would construct at the crown of his head, where the twins were once conjoined. The good news in that regard was that—as anyone who has ever gained a few pounds can tell you—skin expands and grows when it is stretched.

The first surgery would involve the placement of the same kind of skin expanders I had used with Alex Mather—and hundreds of other patients—under each boy's scalp at five separate locations. Once they were surgically implanted, the expanders would be injected with saline solution once each week for the next four months, increasing the bladder's size each time, stretching the boys' skin and allowing it time to grow into its new configuration. Ultimately, we would inject more than a quart of fluid, forming big, elongated "bubbles" along the boys' foreheads and temples, creating at least a hundred square inches of extra skin.

The skin had to be expanded where it was needed; and it had to form flaps that could be peeled back, with one edge left attached to the scalp to maintain a supply of blood, keeping the skin alive during the long separation surgery. The flaps were meticulously designed to ensure that they were well supplied with blood and that they meshed with surrounding tissue and fit together like the pieces of leather that cover a baseball.

Now that separation surgery was planned for the fall, we would need a custom-made surgical table that would function something like a rotisserie, allowing us to rotate the boys 360 degrees during the very lengthy separation procedure and to access the entire circumference of their heads without having to lift, turn, and redrape them, which would have added many hours to the surgery. KCI, a San Antonio–based medical technologies company, donated the five-hundred-thousand-dollar table, built to our team's specifications, including a mechanism that would allow us to split the table in two once the separation was completed, enabling two surgical teams to continue their work without disturbing either boy.

Over the course of spring and summer, we would repeatedly practice with life-size models of the boys tucked into the plastic cases that would anchor them to the special table, and with the operating room floor marked with tape to demonstrate the exact positions of vital equipment, instruments,

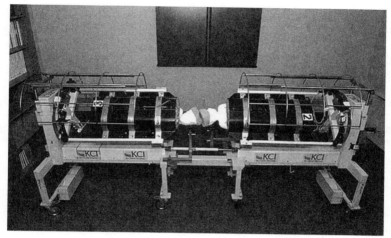

The specially designed operating table for the twins' surgery

and personnel. It was during those early dry runs that the two teams of anesthesiologists, who would stand at each boy's head at opposite ends of the table, realized that the room would be so crowded and the noise level so high that they would need walkie-talkies to communicate with one another.

Our practice sessions offered us invaluable information as we began to make final decisions about the planned chain

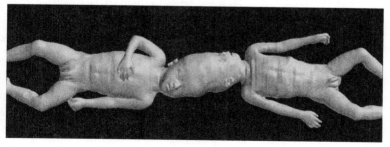

Preoperation model of the Egyptian twins

of events and individual responsibilities, and I know that, like me, each member of our team of more than fifty people began to rehearse in his or her mind the intricate series of procedures that each of us would have to perform perfectly if our ultimate shared goal was to be met.

But first, the skin expanders had to be implanted. Although Ibrahim knew that this procedure was by far the simplest of those that would follow over the next couple of years, he was so nervous on the morning of April 28, 2003, that he could barely speak when I met him before I scrubbed. He told me he would be praying throughout the surgery and I thanked him for that assistance—and for trusting me with his sons.

It had been more than two years since I first had seen a photograph of Ahmed and Mohamed and imagined helping them, and at last I was about to do a bit of the work I had done for more than three decades. In a way I still marvel that after all those years, I was about to take a knife and cut them open in the hope of making them whole.

At Medical City Dallas that day, we inserted five tissue expanders in the twins' heads and one in the lateral thigh of each of their legs—a total of nine expanders that a few months later would produce the tissue to provide the critical watertight seal for their brains and skin for their scalps when we ultimately closed their heads after the separation surgery. Inserting expanders is a simple procedure, and although nothing about the boys' case was ever truly simple, we placed the expanders precisely where we intended to and without any complications. Planning for and providing enough vascularized tissue for a watertight seal is one of the keys to every successful separation surgery—and its absence had been a principal reason for failure in a number of previous cases.

I would place threaded metal pins in predetermined spots in the boys' cheekbones just before the separation surgery, pins that would provide anchorages to which a custom-designed lightweight circular head brace would be attached around each boy's head. At the beginning of the separation surgery itself, we would superficially place a third pin in the base of each boy's skull, but all these maneuvers would have to wait until then because the boys had to lie on the backs of their heads in the meantime.

Once all three pins were linked to the circular head brace as the separation surgery ultimately was under way, the brace, in turn, would be clamped tightly to the rotatable operating bed, ensuring that the boys' heads would not—could not—move even a millimeter during the long hours we knew the surgery would last. But little did I know that day in April, as I focused on every detail of the surgical plan, that six months from then our inability to deeply anchor the third pin at the back of each boy's skull would become a critical and potentially disastrous concern.

During the following months, the nine tissue expanders were very carefully and slowly injected with saline solution to expand the overlying soft tissue; it was essential for us to proceed very delicately to ensure that none of the new tissue was torn or punctured, causing it to die and have to be discarded. Even the smallest issues could have a very large impact on our overall success, and all of us on the craniofacial and pediatric neurosurgical team continued to practice our specific roles virtually every day—particularly once the separation surgery at last was firmly scheduled for Saturday and Sunday, October 11 and 12. We chose to operate on a weekend, when everyone could clear their schedules and plan to be at Dallas Children's Medical Center for as many as forty-eight hours, and at a time of the week, too, when the hospital itself would be at its quietest.

In planning meetings, I had encouraged the nine surgeons, six scrub nurses, eight anesthesiologists, and two dozen other support personnel not only to visualize in minute detail each step of their role in the separation surgery—just as many top athletes and performers do—but also to visualize repeatedly our success, asking them to imprint pictures, even movies, in their minds of Ahmed and Mohamed sitting up, standing, walking, smiling, happy—and separate.

I believed it was essential for all of us to bring positive intention to the operating room as yet one more tool to help us perform at peak levels and also to help balance the inevitable concerns each of us harbored. I personally remained extremely concerned about what the outcome would be. Would there be sufficient venous drainage for the boys' brains once they were separated? Would we have enough tissue to close their brains and seal them off from possible infection? How successfully would the leg fascia grafts function as brain lining, and would pressure inside the twins' brains be normal? Would the boys recover in ways we assumed they would?

We knew their motor cortexes were interlocked like the fingers of two clasped hands and that as a result, both boys initially would have some degree of muscle weakness on one side of their bodies. But because children's brains have the remarkable ability to renew and regenerate neurological

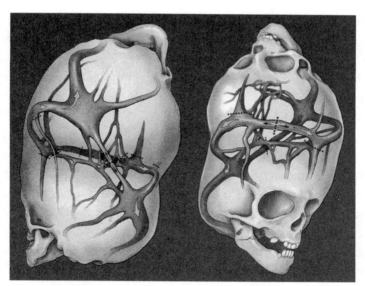

A venous model of the conjoined twins

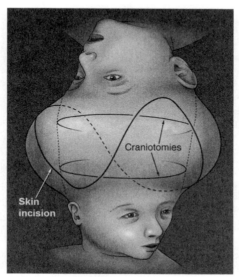

A diagram of the twins' surgical plan

pathways, we believed they had strong potential for overcoming this problem or adapting to the weakness. But what if the resulting neurological deficits were severe? This possibility and a hundred others whirled through my mind constantly, and I thought about virtually nothing else on the long night before surgery.

I was deeply concerned about the possibility that the boys would not survive the surgery. Yet at the same time, I had an abiding sense that we had formulated a brilliant plan to separate them, that we were extremely well prepared, and that we absolutely were doing the right thing. Separation surgery was the only hope Mohamed and Ahmed had for any sort of normal life—and instead of sleeping or incessantly worrying on that Friday night before the surgery commenced, I calmed myself and settled my nerves simply by envisioning them leading wonderful lives.

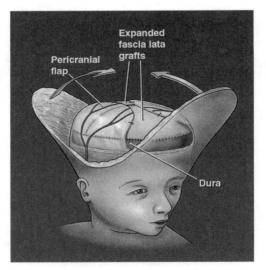

A diagram of the postseparation plan

Chapter Nine

Face to Face

Late in the afternoon of Saturday, October 11, 2003, I made the initial incision into the conjoined scalps of Ahmed and Mohamed Ibrahim, and the separation surgery we had planned and anticipated for so long was under way. But before I raised my scalpel, I suggested to the assembled team—now poised to begin the most complex single surgery of our lives—that if we were ultimately successful in separating the boys, it would be premature to cheer or celebrate in any way until days or weeks afterward, when a true measure of our accomplishment would be clearer, when we would know whether, in fact, we *had* succeeded.

With my initial cuts, I created the first of several skin flaps that would be absolutely essential when, dozens of hours later, we would need to suture them together to cover the boys' separated skulls and brains. The tissue expanders that months before had been placed between their scalps and skulls—now fat with saline solution and almost as large as the boys' heads—were simple to remove, but then it was time to open their skulls. Drs. Ken Shapiro and Dale Swift led a team of five pediatric neurosurgeons, cutting out windows of bone from the backs of the boys' skulls to allow the surgeons to reach their brains. Through these windows, the surgeons slowly and *very* carefully gained access to the boys' combined sagittal sinus and clamped it. When both boys remained stable, we collectively agreed that it was safe to tie off this major venous drainage of the brain and proceed.

Step by meticulous step, we dissected the boys' brains, the neurosurgeons taking the lead, normally working two at a time and often using microscopes to ensure that their work was precise. Throughout the long night, the children were rotated in their special bed, turned incrementally each time to allow us to cut away more skull, expose more brain, and separate Ahmed's brain tissue from Mohamed's. Each time a piece of bone was removed, we saved it so that as we closed, it could be implanted or "banked" in the boys' inner thighs, where it would remain safe, viable, and alive for a year or so, until we were ready to reconstruct their skulls.

Gradually, and in tiny and painstaking steps, the neurosurgeons separated the boys' brain tissue, clipping a vessel, sealing it, then moving to the next, and peeling the two brains apart, a bit as you would try to separate two photographs that are stuck together without damaging either. In the middle of the night, we discovered to our surprise and real concern that one area, comprising about ten percent of the boys' combined brain mass, was shared between them, which we had not previously understood. Now the neurosurgeons had to make a critical decision about how to separate that section, teasing it apart, providing each boy with his share, cognizant that the shared brain was part of their motor cortex but uncertain, of course, about whether the surgeons' choices—and their decisive cuts—would affect one or both boys' motor control. It was daunting, but it had to be done. And we pressed on.

It was in the early hours of the morning as well when we had to address the large blood-engorged ring that circled the boys' brains and served as their sagittal sinus. In some ways, we had worried more about this ring and the potential for massive blood loss when it was severed and divided than the other obstacles we knew we would face during the entire procedure. But the clamping and tying of smaller vessels that had progressed during the preceding hours served us remarkably well. When neurosurgeons Dale Swift and Bradley Weprin cut into the big vessel, the bleeding they encountered was minimal; we contained it, the boys remained stable, and everyone at the table breathed a sigh of relief.

It wasn't until a bit later when potential disaster suddenly loomed. Every aspect of the surgery was going better than any of us had dared to presume it would; our years of planning were paying off brilliantly. But then, suddenly, the third pin from the metal halo surrounding the boys' skull—the one we'd only been able to secure superficially because of underlying venous danger—came loose, and when it did, the whole of the stabilizing head brace also loosened. The twins' heads, which *had* to remain utterly motionless, now were mobile, if only slightly, and it was a moment of real crisis. Doing my best to remain sterile, I had to fight my way through surgical drapes to reach the loose pin, and then—with my breath held and my focus as intense as if I were disarming a bomb—I worked to secure it to the piece of skull the two boys still shared.

Critical seconds passed; no one moved except me, and

then, quickly, I had it. The pin was tight again; the boys' heads were secure, and we had averted catastrophe. The experience was absolutely hair-raising, but in the end, it was the only moment throughout the long night that engendered great alarm.

By late morning on Sunday, the circumference of the boys' common skull had been cut away; they no longer shared any cranial bone, and the neurosurgeons announced that they were severing the last vestiges of brain that bound the two boys. Word quickly spread among the staff and surgeons who were out of the room on break. Everyone wanted to be present and the OR quickly filled, but there simply wasn't space for fifty or more people, so the hospital video team worked quickly to set up a screen, allowing everyone to observe the moment that had been our goal, in fact our obsession, for so long.

With a sign from the neurosurgeons, engineers from KCI—who had fabricated the table specifically for this single operation—crouched beneath it and began to very carefully loosen the bolts that had held the two halves of the table together. Millimeter by millimeter, the engineers pulled the table apart as the neurosurgeons peeled in two the final bits of gray matter that still linked the boys. Then suddenly, we could see the tiles of the operating room floor through the sliver of space that now separated their brains. With Drs. Shapiro, Weprin, and Barceló and me on Mohamed's side of the table and Drs. Frederick Sklar, Swift, and David Genecov on Ahmed's, the table—now two tables—rotated still farther apart. One bed rolled to the left, the other to the right; each boy was on his own life-support system now; each boy had a team attending solely to him, and for the first time since early in their gestation, Ahmed and Mohamed were no longer conjoined.

There were no congratulations, and no one believed for an instant that our work was done. In fact, there was probably a greater risk for injury at that moment than at any point in the surgery. Both boys' brains were exposed; neither had the top of a skull to protect it, and even the subtle pull of gravity now became a concern.

At 11:37 a.m. on Sunday, October 12, phase one was complete. Much surgery immediately remained to be accomplished, but I nonetheless felt a wave of joy and an elated sense of success. At the very least, these two children were now two entirely different and separate boys, and they were stable, and I dared to hope that in the coming days they would be able to look at each other's faces for the first time in their lives.

As the neurosurgeons completed their tasks, I briefly left the operating room and went to find the boys' parents. They were waiting in a room nearby, accompanied by the boys' Egyptian nurses; my wife, Luci; and Sue Blackwood. When I shared the good news, Ibrahim and Sabah were overwhelmed. "Allah be praised and thanked for this great gift," Ibrahim said. Sabah wept softly; tears of joy filled the eyes of everyone in the room, including my own, but I knew we had many hours of complex work to do before the boys' heads were closed and they were safe, and soon I headed back into the operating room, scrubbed in again, and, with my colleagues, began the layer-by-layer closing of both boys' heads.

Ken Shapiro, Raul Barceló, and I and our assistants focused on Mohamed, whom we thought was more at risk, while Dale Swift, David Genecov, and others worked to close Ahmed's head. As I held Mohamed's brain in my hands, keeping it in place as we turned the high-tech bed into an upright position, chills went down my spine. Both boys were remaining remarkably stable; the anesthesiologists reported that their vital signs were not wavering, and our meticulous plan to cover the boys' brains was under way.

Now we were ready for the tissue we had harvested at the beginning of the surgery, as well as the tissue that had been created by inserting expanders into both boys' thighs back when the scalp expanders were placed. Specifically, we would use the fascia, the fibrous connective tissue that covers the muscles of the thigh, in place of the tough, protective tissue known as the dura that normally rests between the brain and the skull.

My excitement mounted as we prepared the patchwork of expanded fascia from Mohamed's legs and carefully sewed the pieces in position, quilting the tissue together to form a watertight seal and the first layer of closure. I hadn't slept in a very long time, but I had no sense of being tired. My concentration remained acute, but accompanying it now was an unmistakable sense of pleasure as well.

We worked rapidly but exceedingly carefully to stitch the fascia to the existing dura, drape it over Mohamed's brain, and ensure that it was as secure and impenetrable as we could make it. Then it was time to fold the skin flaps into place over the fascia, making sure that they, too, fit perfectly. Each boy would have no protective skull bone at the crown of his head for roughly a year, and although each would wear a helmet during this period, it was vitally important for us to seal their brains to prevent leakage of cerebrospinal fluid and seal out bacteria that could cause infection.

For both boys, this final stage of the separation surgery went as smoothly as we could have hoped, and throughout the entire procedure, one that had lasted thirty-four hours by then, their vital signs remained constant—a testament to the remarkable supporting work of the team of anesthesiologists who monitored them.

At long last, I pulled off my mask and gloves and made my way back to the waiting room to tell the boys' parents that each was doing remarkably well and that both were en route to the pediatric intensive care unit, where they would remain in induced comas for several days to help their bodies adjust to the massive assault they had just endured. I explained to Ibrahim and Sabah that they would be able to visit the boys before long and cautioned them not to be alarmed by all the tubes and wires they would find attached to their sons, explaining that the boys would be taken off respirators and would be able to breathe on their own in a few days. There was much to be thankful for, we privately agreed; the boys were separated and alive and well; but much remained uncertain.

Thousands of people from Dallas to Cairo were eager to hear how the surgery had gone, and the administrators at Dallas Children's Medical Center had scheduled a press conference—the lead surgeons' last obligation of the day. Television networks and newspapers from around the world were covering the event as if it were a moon landing—and the procedure had been as complicated in many ways.

"We're very pleased with the surgical outcome, but postsurgery is very important and will determine the success," Dale Swift announced in a blaze of bright light as the cameras started to roll. "Amazingly, everything seemed to follow the plan fairly well." His neurosurgery colleague, Bradley Weprin, cautioned the reporters that "the most critical thing now is the behavior of the wounds and how well they are going to heal." And in addition to lauding the collective work of our fifty-person team, Ken Shapiro praised the people at KCI, who had created the operating table that rotated 360 degrees and split in two once the boys were separated, precisely as it had been engineered to do. "Without the bed," he insisted, "we wouldn't be having this conference today."

I was happy to let the neurosurgeons handle most of the

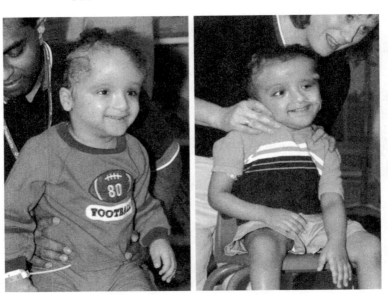

Twins Ahmed and Mohamed following their surgery

questioning; they, after all, had played an extraordinary role in our success, and at last, I could feel a wave of fatigue. I still felt euphoric, but except for a brief nap during the night, I hadn't slept in forty-eight hours, and I realized I was tired. And like everyone else on the team, I knew it was far too soon to pat ourselves on the back or grow complacent. I agreed wholeheartedly with Dr. Jim Thomas, who would be in charge of the boys' care while they remained in the ICU. "Everybody's pulling for these kids," he said, "but they are not out of the woods by any stretch of the imagination."

Soon after the press conference ended, everyone on the team was invited by Luci and me to our home, where we briefly gathered to toast the boys and this successful first stage before we retreated to our beds, where we collapsed into sleep.

A front-page article in the *New York Times* a year before had detailed the twins' plight and the monumental effort under way in Dallas to help them, and Denise Grady, the newspaper's senior medical reporter, was back to cover the surgery, as were reporters from news outlets on several continents. Mike Lorfing, our medical illustrator, ultimately counted more than six hundred stories about the twins in local, national, and international media.

Charlie Gibson and Diane Sawyer at *Good Morning America* did several segments before and after the surgery, and Oprah Winfrey remained fascinated by the work we did in Dallas. Before the boys' surgery, she taped a segment that included an interview with me as well as video of the boys that highlighted the impossibility of their leading normal lives with their heads conjoined at their crowns. And after the surgery, I flew to Chicago for a show with Oprah whose whole hour was devoted to the twins and their successful separation.

Showing photographs and video as we talked in front of Oprah's studio audience, I was able to describe in detail how the two boys spent the first two and a half years of their lives lying on their backs, unable to walk conventionally because of the angle of their attachment. I explained that it had taken over a year for the medical team to come to a decision about whether to separate them, and that we had proceeded believing there was a roughly thirty percent chance that both boys would survive and be fully functioning, because of the complexity of their attachment. "The task seemed almost impossible," I explained to Oprah, "but the boys could have had virtually no quality of life if they had remained conjoined, so we and their parents ultimately decided to attempt the separation."

"Do you feel God used your hand?" Oprah asked at one point.

"Yes, I really do," I responded. "This has been not only a learning experience but a spiritual one as well. No one on this team had ever performed an operation exactly like this. We were guided by a higher power. I think none of us will be the same as a result of having experienced these two little boys."

They were words I profoundly believed. Each of us was blessed to be part of that colossal undertaking, and blessed to have come this far without significant problems. Neither boy had leaked spinal fluid; neither had had an infection. All the flaps and tissue healed nicely, with good vascularity. And most dramatically, the postop CT scans quickly showed that both boys' brains were shifting out of their abnormal shapes and into much more normal configurations—something that seemed almost magical from my point of view, and something that symbolized not only the amazing resiliency of the human body but also the profound rightness of what we had set out to do.

Ahmed and Mohamed left Dallas Children's Medical Center a few weeks after surgery and were transferred back to Medical City Dallas, where they spent the next year in rehabilitation, gradually recovering and receiving tender loving care from dozens of people, including dietitians, physical therapists, psychologists, occupational therapists, and pediatric nurses. With their delightful personalities and endearing eyes, the boys captured the hearts of virtually everyone they encountered. They learned how to sit upright, to stand, and eventually to walk. Ahmed had a number of issues with his gait but eventually could walk using a walker. Within a few months, Mohamed was *running*.

Because the twins had been lying on their backs all of their lives till then, however, their gastrointestinal tracts did not function in a normal fashion once they were upright. The boys were forced to endure feeding tubes in their stomachs for months on end, and ultimately, well more than a year passed before their gastrointestinal tracts assumed normal peristaltic motion and they could begin to eat normally, sitting up.

In addition to ensuring that the twins remained as healthy as possible, we soon began to focus our efforts on the best way to create a new crown for each boy. About the time the separation surgery was completed, we were referred to

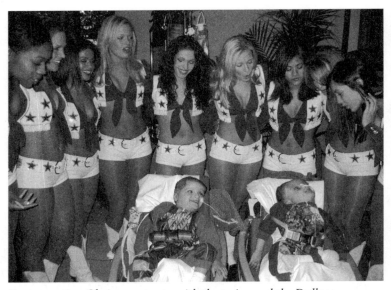

Postoperation Christmas party with the twins and the Dallas Cowboys cheerleaders

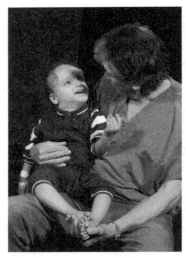

Dr. Salyer with Ahmed

Dane Miller, the CEO at Biomet, a highly successful Indiana company he had cofounded that made innovative products for orthopedics. Dane was a no-nonsense but deeply compassionate entrepreneur who immediately wanted to help us help the boys, and he was quick to focus his company's resources of several kinds toward that end. A stocky, bearded Santa Claus of a guy, he was so captivated by the initial success of the separation surgery and the critical need to give the boys strong skulls that he personally offered one hundred thousand dollars to aid our research in Dallas, as well as ensuring that his researchers in Indiana were always ready to assist us.

Working in concert, we focused our initial attention on a variety of different materials and approaches to the problem, debating whether to fit the boys with prosthetic skulls made of metal or plastic, or to use demineralized bone and other techniques to encourage new growth of natural bone. In the end, it was very clear that real bone would give each boy the best skull—then and far into the future—and we began to work intensively with a solution that would entail the use of demineralized bone, but only as part of an overall framework made out of a resorbable material Biomet had developed—a polyglycolic acid polymer that disappeared after six months, at which time new bone would form within the resorbable framework.

In the research labs at the institute, we performed tests with animals to determine the best method for stimulating bone growth. We would certainly use the curved pieces of the twins' own skull bone that waited in their thighs, but much more additional coverage was needed. We had to decide how to produce it, and our experimental studies

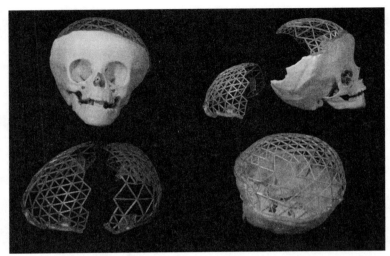

Postsurgical models of skull reconstruction for Ahmed and Mohamed

showed us that the best way was to use a geometric design with resorbable material forming a latticework into which we would insert demineralized bone segments as well as bone morphogenic protein. This method would allow each boy to regenerate his own skull with bone from his own stem cells and osteoblasts. We were embarking on something utterly new in the separation of twins joined at the head, and we were aware as we planned that our work with the twins would provide an important step in improving the technological approach to the separation of conjoined twins around the world.

We had waited well over a year by the time we were ready to schedule the first of the two skull surgeries. Ahmed and Mohamed had needed that time to fully heal, and their brains especially needed time to completely recover from the insult of such a massive operation. But the truth was that we had also needed that time to be sure we were choosing the very best method possible by which to provide them with new skulls.

Several challenges had to be addressed, and most importantly, we needed to complete the skull reconstruction in a single surgery. The boys' brains just couldn't be expected to endure a series of additional assaults. Our goal was simply to give both skulls solid coverage to provide protection for these very active boys for the rest of their lives and allow them to return to Egypt and lead normal lives.

I'd had good experience with demineralized bone in many different skull replacement cases over the years. But I had almost exclusively used it for replacement of skull at a donor site, using the patient's natural bone as the primary replacement in critical areas where skull bone was missing. The scaffold design was an entirely new concept, one that involved creating a geometric latticework of interconnected tiny triangles, fabricated from the resorbable material and shaped individually for each boy's head. Dozens of little triangles of demineralized bone then would be fitted into each triangular opening in the framework.

We knew from our own experience in craniofacial surgery that children at Mohamed's and Ahmed's age can never totally regenerate protective-quality skull to the extent that it's needed. Our job, therefore, was to guide and assist their bodies in regenerating new skulls by stimulating and directing the new growth into a shape and configuration that we could control. What we were planning was in situ bioengineering; we would stimulate their basic stem cells to become osteoblasts, directing new bone into the skull shape we wanted by providing the matrix and shape of the new skull.

I performed Ahmed's reconstruction surgery—the first of the two—in February 2005, sixteen months after the separation. His operation came first because he needed less overall reconstruction than Mohamed did, and also because he was regenerating bone in a much better fashion and at a better rate than his brother. Ahmed's surgery would be less challenging, to some degree, and something of a trial run before we attempted Mohamed's reconstruction.

On a CT scan, we could see before the surgery that Ahmed had done a great job of regenerating new bone from the edges of the base of his skull during the year we waited. When I observed that regrowth firsthand once his skull was exposed in the operating room, I made a quick, but I think shrewd, decision to abandon the plan to employ the synthetic latticework in favor of using solely his own cranial bone, which had been stored in his thigh during the separation surgery.

Sixteen months before, we had circumferentially cut away a big, wide band of bone around the conjoined boys' skull—now a collection of pieces approximately an inch and a half to two inches wide by two and a half to three inches long—to allow us to gain access to their brains. And when I saw to my surprise how very well Ahmed was creating new skull, as well as how much of his own bone was available, the decision to simply use that bone as the matrix for new bone formation was a simple one.

I arranged the segments of bone as if they were puzzle pieces, tying them together with resorbable thread to create a bony crown for Ahmed's head—one with holes in it, yes, but holes that his body would naturally fill with new bone over time. To help stimulate that new growth, I also implanted bone morphogenetic protein at strategic sites. This naturally occurring growth factor was officially approved only for use in repairing fractures of long bones and spurring intervertebral disk regeneration, but I was confident, based on my research and personal experience, that it stood a good chance of stimulating cranial bone growth as well, and Ahmed's reconstruction surgery was a great success.

In the time since separation, however, Mohamed had not regenerated his skull to the degree we would have liked. Based on preoperative studies, I felt certain that he would need the entire scaffold we had planned and fabricated for him, as well as the many triangles of demineralized bone with which we would fill it.

When we exposed the upper part of Mohamed's brain a few weeks after Ahmed's surgery, it was gratifying to see how well he was healing overall, despite the fact that the new growth of skull bone was lagging a bit. That was acceptable, because in his case, the new framework that would hold the triangular demineralized bone was the perfect solution. CT scans and 3-D models had made it possible for the synthetic latticework to be the precise size and shape we needed, allowing me simply to secure it to the natural bone at the base of Mohamed's skull by drilling holes and placing sutures to hold it tightly in place.

The scaffolding fit smoothly over the neo-dura we had created from fascia in Mohamed's thigh more than a year before—we didn't have to expose or disturb his brain again.

Then I meticulously sutured dozens of triangles of demineralized bone into the holes in the framework. The crown of Mohamed's head looked a lot like a geodesic dome by the time we were finished. It looked terrific, in fact, and in his case as well, I implanted a collagen sponge of bone morphogenetic protein—equally convinced, as I was with Ahmed, that it would spur bone growth and the knitting together of all the triangular pieces over the next year or two.

The completion of the second skull reconstruction surgery was a great moment. Both operations—although quite different from each other in the end—had gone as well as we could have hoped. Just as Ahmed had, Mohamed recovered quickly from his second surgery, and sure enough, just a few months later CT scans proved that both boys were generating new skull bone at a rapid pace.

Separation and reconstruction of the skulls of these marvelous boys formed the pinnacle of my career in many ways. The separation surgery necessitated levels of teamwork and commitment to success that were extraordinary. And the reconstruction was also a triumph, the product of forty years of research dedicated to finding the very best ways to create bone or support bone regeneration. Together, the surgeries involved taking many techniques that had been advanced by research and clinical experience around the world and combining them to achieve successful separation and reconstruction with closure and new skulls, as well as ensuring that both boys had aesthetically acceptable faces and heads by the time their medical odyssey was complete.

For me personally, the foremost challenge was not the technical execution of any single surgical aspect of what

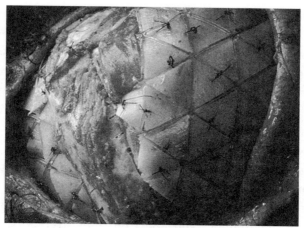

Mohamed's skull reconstruction graph during surgery

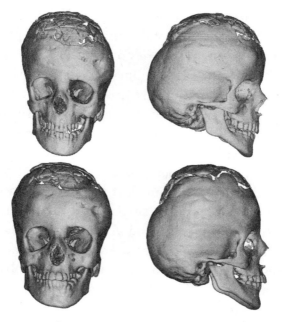

Skull regeneration after operation plan

was done, or of all of them in combination. Throughout my career, I'd faced a number of more challenging situations that had to be solved in the operating room at the moment they presented themselves. With Mohamed and Ahmed, the greatest hurdles had to be gotten over long before we finally rolled the still-conjoined boys in for surgery. The greatest trials were in planning, leading, coordinating, and motivating a team of such magnitude toward such a specific goal, as well as confronting the mountain of ethical, administrative, and financial issues that arose along the way.

The twins' case necessitated the development of new methods, techniques, and research data over a two-year period to create an immensely complex step-by-step plan, and called for more than fifty individuals to execute the plan to the utmost of their professional abilities. For me, the case offered a wonderful example of what plastic surgery has always been—a series of challenges that stimulate new, creative solutions and ultimately offer our patients better lives—and I think most reconstructive plastic surgeons would agree that that's why the subspecialty is so attractive.

Every case is different, of course, yet the goal is always the same: providing quality of life and a close approximation of normalcy for young people whose lives otherwise would be dramatically limited, if not simply thin shadows of life. Without separation surgery and the reconstruction that followed, Mohamed and Ahmed would have never walked, never stood, never looked at each other face to face; their lives would have been very narrow and probably very short. But the collective work on two continents—without any consideration given to distinctions between cultures and religions—to give them good lives was a metaphor, I feel, for how people inherently want to build human brotherhood and move toward a higher consciousness, recognizing that when we bring joy to one life, to two, we bring joy to all of humankind.

In the first years after the terrible events of September 11, 2001, it was wonderfully gratifying—and really humbling—to observe Americans by the thousands embracing these two helpless and innocent Muslim boys and coming to their rescue. The World Craniofacial Foundation ultimately received more than a million dollars in donations specifically earmarked for the care and treatment of Ahmed and Mohamed. Total in-kind, donated, and billed costs for their great adventure in the United States reached nearly four million dollars in the end, yet everything that was offered to the boys came freely, given with nothing more than love and hope for bright futures for both boys.

That level of concern and support, I believe, demonstrated then and continues to demonstrate years later that deep in our hearts, we *know* we are all part of the same family, that each of us possesses something extraordinary that we call the human spirit—perhaps because we have no better words—and that God, indeed, is love.

Mohamed and Ahmed helped me personally understand those truths in ways I never had before. Their gift to me and many of our team members was a wonderful new cognizance of soul connectedness and the purpose of individuals' lives. Once more, the two boys confirmed for me that I had made exactly the right decision when I became a physician long ago and learned to heal children physically trapped by facial deformity.

As Deepak Chopra has pointed out, the soul is not in

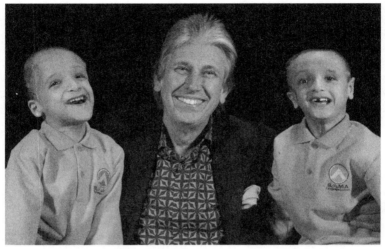

Dr. Salyer with Ahmed and Mohamed

the body, but the body is in the soul. Each of us profoundly needs our body to live a full and rich and soulful life, and it has been my great reward, my blessing, to provide young people like Ahmed and Mohamed with bodies that allow them to pursue their spirits' missions.

In thousands of newspaper articles and television news stories in every corner of the world, people learned about these two boys, their terrible plight and their triumph, and people's hearts were opened so widely that they could never close tightly again. I've always been struck by the fact that virtually every one of the world's major religions includes among its tenets the idea that we should treat those around us as we wish to be treated. It's apparently a universal notion, and it does seem to represent our highest human ideal.

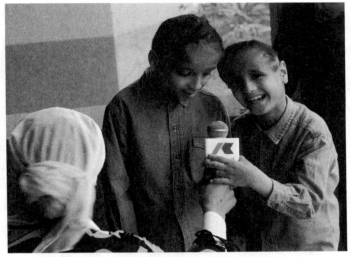

Separated twins Ahmed and Mohamed during an interview

In ways both simple and profound, thousands of people chose to give the two boys the literal and metaphorical freedom they wanted for *their* children and themselves. And in return, the boys opened their hearts to the wonderful ways in which giving becomes receiving and spreading love guarantees its receipt.

In November 2005, it was time at last for the boys to return to Egypt, where their brother and sister and extended family eagerly awaited them. They had been in Dallas for three and a half years; both spoke fluent English as well as Arabic now, both were continuing to recover remarkably successfully, and both continued to captivate our hearts. To celebrate their return home, the World Craniofacial Foundation hosted a farewell party for the boys at the C. R. Smith

Museum in nearby Fort Worth, with American Airlines providing the venue and all the costs associated with the celebration as a gift to the boys. More than two hundred people attended, including many who had performed critical roles during the thirty-four-hour separation surgery and many more who had helped treat and care for the boys throughout their long Texas sojourn.

It was a great afternoon; the spirit of true celebration seemed to fill the cavernous space and lift all of us off our feet—and it was an emotional day for me as well. I would see the boys again, of course—both in Egypt and on their return to Dallas. But this was a festive day we could not

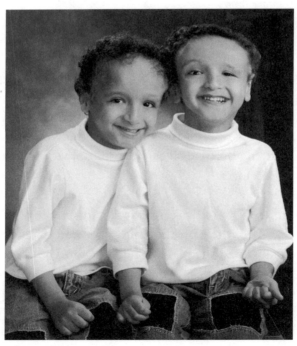

A recent photo of the twins

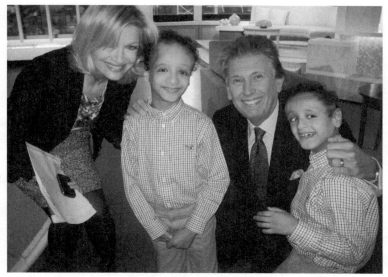

The twins, Ahmed and Mohamed, with Diane Sawyer

have dared to presume was on the horizon back when they first arrived. Nor could I have known long ago when I, too, was a sick child in real need of help that one day I would realize my spiritual connectedness to others and to God by caring for patients like these as a physician and a surgeon.

These little boys entered my life at a time when they needed a miracle. They received it, in the end, but it was a miracle that came for *all* of us to share and savor.

Chapter Ten

Change, Reflection, Resolve

During a trip to Japan in 1999 to give a keynote lecture to the Japanese Society of Oral and Maxillofacial Surgeons, I noticed some numbness in my left foot. It persisted throughout the trip, and I couldn't make sense of what it was or what might have caused it.

I returned home and dove back into my hectic schedule and did my best to ignore the strange and irritating lack of feeling, but when it continued to be bothersome several months later, I went to see a neurologist at Medical City who examined me, did nerve conduction and other studies, then sat me down in his office to tell me that I was suffering the onset of "cryptogenic idiopathic peripheral neuropathy." In other words, somewhere outside my brain or spinal cord I had damaged nerves, but it was unclear precisely where the damage was and what had caused it.

It wasn't a diagnosis I wanted to hear, and it didn't help when the young neurologist—to whom I'd been recommended because he had a great reputation—added that he simply didn't know whether the numbness would get worse or whether it would spread. "Something like this frequently turns out to be a symptom of some underlying cancer or other disease," he continued, and by then the wind had gone completely out of my sails.

I was a guy who worked on his feet, for heaven's sake, and I planned to keep working for a good long while, and the possibility of living with diffuse numbness or *cancer* was a thought I wasn't eager to entertain. I didn't panic— I'd been around medicine long enough to need a lot more information before it was time to panic, if ever—but the diagnosis was worrisome.

The neurologist scheduled a complete workup and assessment and ultimately found no immunologic or other etiologic cause for the neuropathy. I received a clean bill of health overall, but the numbness persisted, so he referred me to a neurologist at the University of Texas's Southwestern Medical School, the location of my general surgery residency, and my former employer. Dr. Gil Wolfe was an expert in peripheral neuropathy, and, it turned out, he and my son, Ken, Jr., had known each other in high school; although he seemed like a great young guy, he gave me some stunning information on the heels of further testing and evaluation.

"You do, indeed, have a neuropathy," he concluded. It would progress at an unknown rate, maybe quickly, maybe slowly. It might spread to my hands and upper extremities, and it could eventually affect my motor system and cause paralysis. The bottom line of his very bad news was that he was convinced I had a progressive neurological disorder that would inevitably take me on a downhill course that would change my life dramatically. *Now* it was time to panic.

Besides the herniated lumbar disk I suffered when I was

a plastic surgery resident at the University of Kansas School of Medicine, which was serious enough that I had to have a laminectomy and which caused me to fail my air force physical, I'd had other significant medical problems over the years related to the thousands of hours I spent at the operating table. In the early 1980s, I had to have two cervical vertebrae fused and a bone spur removed that was pressing on my spinal cord—injuries I believed were caused by years of wearing a heavy headlamp on my forehead during surgery and standing in abnormal positions for long hours. After that operation, I was unable to work for three months and had to wear a cervical collar around my neck to keep that part of my spine immobile. It was uncomfortable and inconvenient—and not working for three months drove me slightly mad—but I knew that with a bit of patience I would improve and be able to return to my normal schedule and to the operating room.

But this time, my diagnosis was *very* different. This time, it appeared I would never improve and, in fact, might well lose not only my capability to perform surgery but also my ability to walk. I was only sixty-four years old and hadn't begun to consider retiring, but the neuropathy and the numbness in my feet were worsening with each week, each month, and suddenly my future appeared utterly changed.

Initially, I told very few people and did my best to move forward as if all were well. My energy wasn't affected in any way; I didn't experience numbness in any other part of my body; my acuity with my hands remained as keen as ever and my surgical skills did not diminish. Yet now there was always the nagging awareness in my mind that my body was in the early stages of betraying me and that it was very possible, perhaps even probable, that one day soon I would no longer be able to work as a surgeon—the only work I'd ever done and work that I continued to deeply love.

The extraordinary era of the 1990s and everything that had coalesced to bring the institute into existence and allow us to create what we believed was the finest comprehensive craniofacial center in the world began to shift into a new form about the time I developed the peripheral neuropathy. Although the two circumstances were unrelated, their combined impact on me was weighty enough that I had to begin to confront the truth that nothing is constant and that change is a fundamental component of any endeavor, and of life itself.

My partner and fellow craniofacial surgeon Ian Munro surprised all of us at the institute when in 1994 he announced his retirement at the young age of sixty. Our neurosurgery colleague Derek Bruce retired seven years later, in 2001. Then Ken Shapiro, the second pediatric neurosurgeon on our team, decided to retire not long after we had separated the Egyptian twins. I understood their decisions, but I hated to see them go. We'd created something unique, something remarkable, at the institute, and each of them had been vital to its success. They were men who had grown eager to spend quality time with wives and children and grandchildren at long last, eager to dive into other passions like skiing, fly-fishing, sailing, and golf while they were still fit and healthy. And they were ready, too, to be honest, to flee the changes in contemporary medicine that had begun to disillusion doctors everywhere—most particularly the advent of "managed care" and the increasing supremacy of health insurance companies over physicians in the realm of patient treatment.

The Institute for Craniofacial and Pediatric Neurosurgery was very well established after a decade and a half. It had become world renowned, and we were doing work that made us proud—transforming the lives of our young patients and moving our subspecialties forward. Derek, Ian, and I—the three principals—traveled widely to speak to other surgeons and consult on specific cases, and each of us had established fellowships, mentoring the generation of craniofacial surgeons and pediatric neurosurgeons who would follow us.

I had directed a craniofacial fellowship since 1979, one

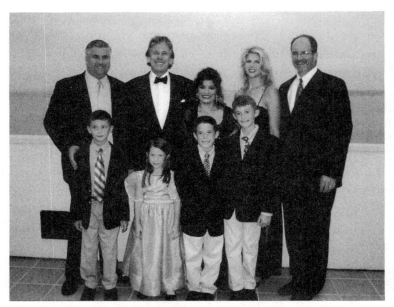

Dr. Salyer with his family in 2003 as president of the International Society of Craniofacial Surgery, Monterey, California

that now was sponsored directly by the World Craniofacial Foundation and approved by the Accreditation Council for Graduate Medical Education. I was proud of its tenure and success; I had become a fine surgeon specifically because of the mentoring I had received from the best reconstructive plastic surgeons in the world, and I believed it was my responsibility to mentor young surgeons in return. Two of my fellows, David Genecov and Raul Barceló, had joined us permanently at the institute, and my dream was that one or both would lead it after my retirement, which, it suddenly appeared, might have to come far sooner than I wanted.

But things *were* changing at Medical City and throughout the health services world, and from my perspective—like those of my retired colleagues—it was hard to believe that they were changing for the better. The remarkable years of support we had received from Humana came to an end in 1992, when Humana sold its hospitals nationwide to the healthcare company HCA and entered the health insurance business. On the heels of the purchase, the hospital—and all of us at Medical City—endured a parade of seven or eight CEOs, each one with a differing management style, set of priorities, and perspective on the value of the craniofacial institute.

Inevitably, perhaps, administrative support for our work softened significantly and funding began to be cut. The clinical team, the research, and the academic environment we had created all suffered, as did our ability to take on charity cases, which had been one of the institute's hallmarks from the beginning. We had never had to turn away a patient because of inability to pay during the Humana era, but now the landscape was very different. Fewer and fewer indigent patients—even those with life-threatening issues—were approved for surgery each year, the numbers dwindling very distressingly until 2005, when Petero Byakatonda became the last charity patient I personally was able to treat at Medical City Dallas. Soon thereafter, no more charity cases were ever approved by the administration.

The institute we had planned, developed, and created now was gradually eroding—bit by bit, but inexorably. The things we foremost had stood for in the beginning— excellence of care, willingness to take on the most challenging cases, creation of an academic center that undertook important translational research, mentoring of the next generation of surgeons, and publishing our latest information in the medical literature—were increasingly complex enterprises because medical care in the United States was changing dramatically, and so were its practitioners.

"Managed care," a variety of administrative techniques intended to reduce the cost of providing health benefits and improve the quality of care, was an idea that didn't work from the outset. Managed care managed money—almost always to the benefit of the insurance companies rather than patients—but it didn't manage medical care. It added bureaucracy and expense, and the old fee-for-service system disappeared. Instead of decreasing costs, medical care in the United States became ever more expensive, to the point that it currently consumes eighteen percent of our gross domestic product, the highest percentage of any nation in the world.

Through no particular fault of their own, the generation of young surgeons then in their thirties and forties found themselves in a medical world that had grown far more complex administratively than it had been twenty or thirty years before, and earning a good living as a surgeon had become more difficult as well.

In the early days at the institute, the reputations of the lead surgeons had been of foremost importance in our ability to attract patients. Children and parents with serious medical issues came to see me, or Dr. Bruce, or Dr. Shapiro, because our reputations were stellar, not because we worked where we happened to work. And when a patient with a fibrous dysplasia tumor of the orbit and face, for example, came to see me, I would likely encounter optic nerve compression, so I would jointly plan treatment and procedures with my neurosurgery colleagues across the hall and would operate alongside them. Three or more of us would work together to achieve outcomes that were better than any of us could have accomplished alone and would often create improved methods and techniques, which we shared with colleagues worldwide.

But as the managed-care era began to alter the medical landscape in dramatic ways, physicians and surgeons were less and less able to be creative or bold. Their rewards were fewer, and the younger generation was far less willing than we had been to push the innovative envelope, opting instead to perform only the procedures they had been taught or were comfortable with and declining to take on the very patients who needed them most. Because the younger surgeons were more constrained by administrative red tape and were therefore less experimental, their successes were more limited and they did not become as well known. They did not teach, travel to meetings to present cases, or write articles about their techniques, methods, and advancements as prolifically as we had. And for all those reasons, they began to attract fewer patients, and revenues fell.

It was an increasingly challenging time for me personally. The numbness in my foot grew steadily worse; close colleagues and dear friends who were my age or even younger had retired or announced their plans to retire; I was increasingly concerned about the institute's future under the banner of HCA; and like thousands of physicians and surgeons around the country, I was ever more disillusioned with the way medicine had to be practiced when insurance companies held far more power than doctors did.

In the mid-1990s, I'd been invited to Saudi Arabia, where I met Crown Prince Sultan. He and I liked each other; we communicated directly and clearly, and we had extensive conversations not only about improving craniofacial care for children in his country but also about the possible development of a joint venture in far north Dallas, where we would build a fifty-million-dollar facility for the treatment of children with surgically treatable congenital, acquired, traumatic, degenerative, and other craniofacial problems.

It was an enormously exciting prospect, one that would allow us to treat one free patient for every paying patient and still operate in the black, based on then-current statistical models. Given the changing medical climate nationally and the institute's uneasy relationship with HCA, I believed this new hospital would allow us to rectify a number of problems and allow me to further the dream we had made a reality with Ira Korman and Humana back in 1986, but which now was rapidly disappearing.

As I envisioned it, this new hospital could even serve as a model for health care throughout the country, one demonstrating that foundation-owned hospitals implementing a dedicated team approach and very high efficiency could successfully care for a specialty group of patients within our society. It was a humanitarian model that would provide free care for indigent patients and still operate in the black, so long as all its employees refrained from being greedy.

Long ago, the Mayo Clinic had been founded as a not-for-profit integrated-care and research institution, one administered by doctors and staffed by doctors from every specialty with a high level of expertise. Over the years, the people at Mayo proved impressively that a hospital run by visionary physicians *can* create a highly efficient and patient-focused product and still thrive financially. The only downside to the model is that the top doctors cannot earn as much money as physicians can at for-profit institutions—it's as simple as that. But I was certain that I could staff a new craniofacial and pediatric neurosurgery hospital with the quality people with whom I'd already been working for years, and pay them well; and instead of also creating profits for shareholders, we would provide excellent care for patients who could not pay.

Working closely with consultants in several fields, we moved forward at a brisk pace, and I was optimistic that with the backing of the prince we would succeed in bringing this new vision to life, just as we had years before with Humana. We had an impressive financial pro forma in place; I found a great parcel of land and was ready to purchase it; we had commissioned preliminary architectural plans for the hospital itself, and had a handshake commitment from Crown Prince Sultan for twenty-five million dollars in initial funding.

But then, rather suddenly, the crown prince turned his attention elsewhere and delegated my dealings with him to Saudi intermediaries. The ease and rapidity with which we had moved till now was replaced on the Saudi end not only with bureaucratic chaos but with bald-faced corruption as well. The people I now had to deal were very clearly bent on making sure that much of the crown prince's money went into their own pockets, and I was faced with a difficult decision. Would I accept Saudi vice and exploitation as the price of achieving yet another dream?

In the end, my conclusion was rather easy, and I walked away, firm in the belief that life was too short to have to work with nefarious partners—no matter what the goal—and cognizant that I had many other important things to do, even if my neuropathy meant that I would have to quit performing surgery. If I had to retire from the institute in the midst of uncertain change, I still could focus my talents on the work of the World Craniofacial Foundation, lecture, teach, and write. Integrity had become an important virtue in my life, and becoming an ally of corrupt and difficult people simply was not an option.

With change whipping at the institute like the flames of a prairie fire, I found not only that I could no longer treat difficult-case patients in the numbers I was committed to, but also that it was becoming increasingly hard to support our twenty-one-person office staff. A partial solution—yet not one I was eager to acquiesce to—seemed to be the development of a cosmetic surgery center as a parallel enterprise.

I certainly supported aesthetic plastic surgery from both a medical and a patient perspective, and I'd done some of it myself over the years. It wasn't a field that ignited my passion, but I understood that as a booming part of the medical industry, cosmetic surgery could help financially support the institute and its employees in very valuable ways.

I was sympathetic, too, to the young surgeons with whom I was working. Given the current state of medicine in the United States, it would increasingly become impossible for them to provide for themselves and their families and their clinical and clerical staffs, travel to meetings, teach, lecture, write textbooks, publish peer-reviewed articles, and advance the subspecialty by treating solely craniofacial and cleft patients. They would *have* to practice cosmetic surgery, at least part-time, to generate enough money to retain their focus on reconstructive plastic surgery.

Reimbursement by Medicaid and Medicare, managed-care health systems, and others was rapidly ratcheting down resources for all types of reconstructive surgery. And it was forcing gifted young surgeons trained to perform state-of-the-art craniofacial work to focus their attention in other areas simply to make a living. It was a reality that I had to accept and do my best to combat in whatever creative ways I could conceive, but it left me concerned foremost for the hundreds of thousands of children who—because of that reality—would not receive the care that would give them a chance in life.

When I trained in medicine and then went into plastic surgery, the medical world was moving from an era of generalization to one of specialization. The decades-old role of the so-called general practitioner was increasingly being

replaced by multiple physicians specializing in internal medicine, pediatrics, gynecology and obstetrics, and other fields.
In the surgical world, general surgery—once the pinnacle of
the art—was being replaced by orthopedic, cardiac, neurological, plastic, and other surgical subspecialties. With more
and more specialization, the general fund of knowledge
inevitably expanded—and that was a good thing.

But the downside of that specialization is the way it limits
a surgeon's skills, making it more difficult for him or her
to treat patients across a spectrum of disorders. And something similar was under way in plastic surgery in the early
2000s, with surgeons splintering their expertise into microsurgery, hand surgery, burn reconstruction, and craniofacial
surgery, and there was increasing pressure to practice either
aesthetic *or* reconstructive surgery, but not both. More and
more plastic surgeons responded to that pressure by opting
to practice solely aesthetic surgery because it offered greater
financial security.

My richly rewarding career had allowed me to earn a
good living out on a new surgical frontier. It was a marvelous opportunity that I and a few others around the world
had fully embraced, shaping craniofacial surgery into a subspecialty that changed lives in a direct and deeply satisfying
way. But as I entered my fourth decade as a plastic surgeon,
I worried that in addition to being attracted by the promise
and fascination of reconstructive surgery, too many young
surgeons were choosing plastic surgery because of a certain
lifestyle it seemed to ensure. Would they venture out and
explore new frontiers, such as finding ways to successfully
perform partial or full transplantations of the face and—an

even loftier goal—to spur the regeneration of patients' own missing body parts?

I believed there would always be a core group of surgeons driven by the desire to help others by breaking new ground and dramatically moving medicine forward. I was sure of it because I still encountered and worked closely with young surgeons who possessed the passion and spirit of discovery and adventure that had filled me at their age. Yet what was increasingly concerning was the possibility that the billowing costs of health care and the complexities of medical practice would make their efforts far more difficult than the

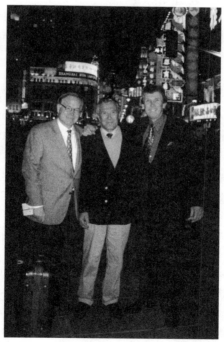

Dr. Salyer with colleagues Bryan Toth and Daniel Marchac in Shanghai

challenges my pioneering colleagues and I had faced several decades before.

It's axiomatic, I suppose: one gift of growing older is your ability to take some stock of your life, its highs and lows, its trajectory and its destination, the ways in which it has mattered so far, and those things you want to make sure you accomplish while you can. For me, an enormous source of pleasure and satisfaction as I began to age was watching a number of patients about whom I cared a great deal become adults and create lives of their own that mattered—to themselves, to their communities, and to those with whom they shared their talents.

Michael Hatfield's road, for example, has not been an easy one to travel, but it's one that has taken him far beyond his simple boyhood desire to have a normal face. As with so many of my patients, Michael's transformation has gone far beyond his series of surgeries and the resulting physical changes they brought him. His challenges—and his successes—became the catalyst for advocacy in support of political and insurance initiatives to improve the lives of thousands of others struggling to resolve craniofacial abnormalities.

Laurie Hatfield remembers that her son, born in 1978 in Houston, "seemed fine to me at first. Then, at about six months, he started becoming agitated all the time—as if he were uncomfortable in his own skin." As Michael matured, his head grew significantly faster than the rest of his body and his eyes began to grow far apart and appeared to be literally sinking into his head.

"I just knew something was horribly wrong, but no one

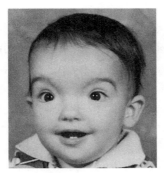

Presurgery photo of Michael Hatfield

could tell me what it was. I even thought about Down's syndrome, but no one would tell me for sure. It was a mother's nightmare. Eventually, Michael had a CT scan, and the diagnosis was hydrocephaly."

"Don't get too attached to the little guy," a doctor told his parents. "Not too much we can do about this, I'm afraid."

Horrified by what they heard from the blunt physician, Laurie and her husband, Jim, nonetheless grew more determined to find a way to help their son. "First, we prayed," she recalls. "We had an amazingly dedicated group of friends, and they joined us in prayer. And, as it turned out, one of my friends had an acquaintance who knew Dr. Linton Whitaker, a renowned plastic surgeon in Pennsylvania."

Laurie wrote to my decadeslong craniofacial colleague and good friend, and he, in turn, suggested they come see me in Dallas. Michael was almost two when I first saw him, and I was able to assure his parents on that first visit that he had been misdiagnosed. His syndrome was frontonasal dysplasia with hypertelorism, I explained, a disorder that could be countered with surgery to reconstruct his malformed face.

A few months later, I performed a subcranial hyper-telorism correction, narrowing Michael's bulging ethmoid sinuses—air-filled cells inside the ethmoid bone—to allow me to move the orbits of his eyes a normal distance from each other. The surgery was a success, but Laurie's first look at her son following the operation made her worry otherwise. "I expected to see my perfect boy, but I swallowed hard when I saw him postsurgery. He was horribly swollen, and his head looked enormous. He had a hose coming out of his nose. The surgery had lasted twelve excruciating hours, and he had to spend a month in the ICU. It was rough on the little guy, and really hard on us, too."

We performed a secondary soft-tissue correction when Michael was four, including medial canthopexies to bring the corners of his eyes closer together and improve their shape. This time, his parents were better prepared for him to look a little beat-up at first, and within a few months, Michael and his mom and dad were very pleased with his progress. But as happens in some frontonasal dysplasia cases, his sinuses grew too large once more, pushing his right orbit and eye out of position.

Michael was nine when we went back into the operating room, and this time I removed his ethmoid sinuses, something I'd never done before. But this ethmoidectomy proved so successful that in more than a hundred subsequent cases, I included it as part of the primary hypertelorism correction, and it became a widely accepted procedure—Michael and I jointly helping many other children with dramatically wide-set eyes in the process.

Over the years, I performed four major surgeries on Michael; he toughed out each of them, but he grew very

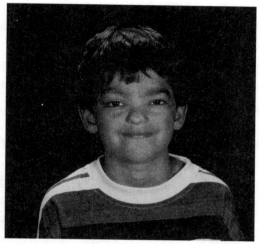

Michael Hatfield postsurgery

weary of doctors and operations at times. When I talked to him not long ago, he still vividly remembered the surgery when he was nine. "I had one complication after another, then a major one that involved a complete rebuilding of my entire face, my nose, and my eye orbits. I was in a lot of pain and I was in grade school, and I got tormented constantly. There was a lot of discrimination during those years. But, then and now, I always tried to remain positive and in the game. I've always relied on humor to get me through challenges."

As Michael reached his high school years, the teasing finally stopped—in part because he now looked remarkably normal but also because he was bright and highly sociable. His parents reported that he had become very outgoing and could make friends easily—and with all kinds of people, too. "It's amazing—he certainly didn't get that from his father or me," his mother told me. "I always thought it was a special, God-given gift to help him get through a life of physical deformities and grueling surgeries."

After Michael's high school graduation, we were just a couple of days from doing what we presumed would be his final surgery when the Hatfields were informed that their insurance company was declining to cover its full cost, claiming it was cosmetic surgery when it absolutely was not. Health Administration Services Inc. of Houston, the plan administrator, would approve payment only for the nasal reconstruction required to improve Michael's breathing. The bulk of the procedure—reshaping his nose and grafting bone to give him stronger cheekbones—would not be covered.

Incensed and incredulous, the Hatfields decided to fight. Laurie confronted the insurance company's top management, and her impassioned appeal ultimately succeeded. The plan administrator agreed to cover all of Michael's surgery, and the company even formally modified its cosmetic surgery exclusion for future patients in Michael's circumstances, sanctioning "cosmetic" surgery for birth defects.

Today, at six feet two inches tall, Michael stands out in any crowd; his height and his gregarious, larger-than-life personality draw people to him—and few even notice anything abnormal about his face. He's an eloquent speaker, and I'm proud of his professional career as a management consultant and the fact that he's recently managed to earn a law degree at the University of Houston Law Center while maintaining a demanding work schedule and active life with his wife, Beth, and sons Sidney and Harrison.

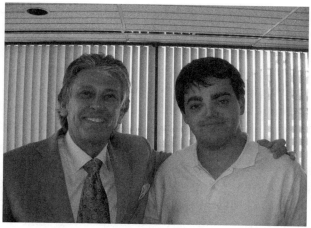

Michael Hatfield following all his surgeries

A few years ago, it was a huge pleasure when Michael joined me on a trip to Washington, DC, where we lobbied on behalf of pivotal legislation to facilitate care for children with craniofacial deformities and guarantee that they cannot be denied coverage for procedures deemed "cosmetic." At the time, countless children were being denied coverage for secondary surgeries they desperately needed—and the struggle continues today.

As part of our presentation before a congressional subcommittee, we screened a video about Michael's life, his medical journey, and his battle for health insurance coverage. He stepped into the congressional spotlight with his trademark energy and enthusiasm, eloquently supporting the need for greater access to surgery for others like him. And although the specific legislation we were supporting did not become law, the experience cemented Michael's commitment to ensuring that children with all kinds of disabilities get the care they need when they need it without bankrupting their families.

Driven by a compelling sense of purpose and an electric spirit, Michael will, I'm sure, always remain focused on what he can do for his family, for children who were born with the same kinds of challenges he was, and for the World Craniofacial Foundation—to which he, like so many of my former patients, offers steadfast support of many kinds.

Michael is no longer my patient; I'm simply honored to call him my friend, and I know I remain important to him as well. The last time we spoke he told me, "I think my partnership with you—and I say that because you've been much more than my surgeon—has helped me a ton in achieving what I have in life. You really wanted me to *have* a life, you felt I deserved one. That was huge. And what a process it's been, just to arrive at 'normal' with you."

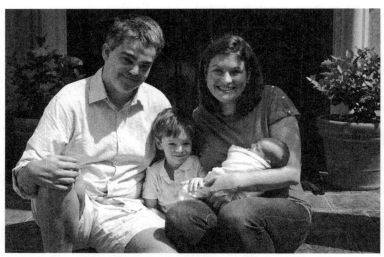

Michael Hatfield as an adult with his family

*   *   *

My neuropathy wasn't becoming dramatically worse, but neither had it disappeared. It remained only sensory for now—affecting sensation in my feet, causing numbness that was disconcerting and worrisome—yet every bit of information I could glean seemed to buttress the diagnosis I had received from neurologist Gil Wolfe: my symptoms would grow worse over time and likely would one day force me out of the operating room.

It was a future I felt I had to face head-on and somehow make the most of, so I made the decision in 2001 to sell my practice but to remain closely allied with it and the institute for five more years—at which time I would turn seventy and, I presumed, be both physically and psychologically ready to leave the operating suites where I had done my work for more than forty years.

Ed Genecov had been my dear friend and colleague for most of those years. A dedicated orthodontist—and a very good one—he was a Dallas native who had played football for Highland Park High School. An always-smiling, genuinely caring, and dedicated family man, Ed was a strong supporter of his local synagogue, and his Jewish faith mattered deeply to him. He and I shared a heartfelt concern for our patients—something that not everyone in the profession brought to his or her work.

Ed was short and stocky; I was tall and lean. I was Don Quixote to his Sancho Panza, and for many years, Ed and I held our own monthly orthodontic and surgical clinic, where we saw new patients, patients who were in preparation for surgery, and follow-up patients. I could never have obtained anywhere near the spectacular results I regularly

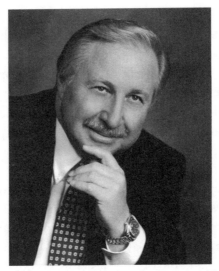

Edward Genecov, Dr. Salyer's friend and colleague of forty years

did with cleft patients and in correcting complex jaw disorders related to structure, growth, and malocclusion without Ed's expertise.

Beginning when he was just sixteen, Ed's only son, David, began to express real fascination with our work, but he seemed more interested in following in my footsteps than his father's—and perhaps Ed urged him in that direction as well. David liked me and I liked him, and I strongly encouraged his interest in craniofacial surgery. Very determined, like his father, David had received his medical degree from the University of Texas at San Antonio and had served residencies in general and plastic surgery at West Virginia University and Wake Forest University. He was my WCF craniofacial fellow in 1995 and 1996, and I know it meant a great deal to his dad—just as it did to me—for us to work together and for David to grow under my tutelage as a very promising young craniofacial surgeon.

I ultimately invited David to come into the practice, and he was joined later by Raul Barceló, a native of Querétaro in central Mexico who had trained in plastic surgery under Dr. José Guerrerosantos at the University of Guadalajara before beginning his fellowship year in Dallas and then permanently joining our team. Raul was a delicate and careful surgeon with a terrific medical knowledge base; he was something of an academic and also an excellent teacher.

I fought hard for Raul to receive a license to practice plastic surgery in Texas—because by the end of his fellowship year I knew I wanted him on our team—but despite my best efforts to help him also get board certified in the United States, that hurdle remained insurmountable. What that meant in practical terms was simply that some potential patients would be wary of his talents, but the fact that he was a valued member of our team largely overcame those concerns.

It was essential, however, for the lead surgeon in the practice to be board certified, so, because I couldn't sell the practice to both David *and* Raul, we created an agreement that would provide David with complete ownership after five years, with Raul technically working for him. I wasn't eager to sell; I'd built something I was proud of, and nothing in me was ready for retirement. But if my continuing health was now suspect—and it was—and if it made sense to begin a new and final phase of my professional career, I was delighted to turn the practice over to David and to continue to work closely with him and Raul for the next five years.

Those were exciting and consequential years. I operated successfully on Petero Byakatonda during that time, and it was the era, too, when we accomplished the near-impossible with the Egyptian twins, Mohamed and Ahmed Ibrahim. The foundation continued to expand its reach and execute its mission to give children everywhere normal faces, and as I continued to perform surgery, travel, teach, and publish without slowing my pace, I also began to imagine—and to set in motion—life beyond the operating room and a time when, like it or not, I would no longer lift a scalpel. Nor would I continue to encounter extraordinary young people who met their disabilities with poise and courage and lend them a vital hand in accomplishing their life's purpose.

Ashley Ashcroft was born in Longview, Texas, in 1982 with a huge hole in the center of her face. She had a complete cleft of her lip and nose as well as of her alveolus, her anterior palate. She had difficulty in swallowing and breathing; talking would be almost impossible for her. I performed my first operation on her when she was just a few months old.

I was one of the pioneers of newborn cleft nasal repair; it had become my signature operation during the initial stages of my career, and it was one I'd improved over the years. Although I was good at virtually every aspect of craniofacial surgery, many of my colleagues around the world would have told you that cleft lip and palate surgeries were my métier, and it would have been difficult for me to argue.

I was taught by David W. Robinson at the University of Kansas not to touch the noses of cleft patients until they were nearly fully grown—the only accepted method in the early 1970s. But once I was operating on my own, I was able to demonstrate that if you performed the surgery *much* earlier, you could achieve significantly better aesthetic results. It was much easier to shape the cartilage of an infant three or four months old than to shape it once the cartilage matured.

Ashley's surgery went very well, and she began to thrive—eating, breathing, and smelling normally, and talking clearly by about eighteen months. We performed secondary refinements on her, doing additional surgery on her lip and nose when she was seven, grafting bone from her hip into the large gap in her upper jaw to create a place for her newly developing teeth to move into and, with the help of orthodontics, giving her beautiful teeth and jaws over time.

Cleft lips and palates are the most frequently occurring congenital deformity of the head and neck region—and that statistic is true around the world. In the United States, the incidence is roughly one in seven hundred births, a ratio that is remarkably similar in countries throughout the developing world. Genetic factors contributing to cleft lip and cleft palate formation remain only partially understood, but it's clear that many types of clefts do run in families.

Ashley was one of about five thousand children with clefts on whom I operated during my career—far more than any other single disorder—and she was representative of so many children I treated who had the good fortune to be supported by a medical team who cared about her not only professionally but also personally. And it was easy to treat children like Ashley as if they were my own. In every case, I strove to produce perfection, just as I would have wanted with my own kids, and that attitude instilled great confidence in me in most of my patients' parents. They believed that I wanted as much for their children as they did, and that made us allies in ways that served everyone.

Ashley's parents were both attractive people—her mother was a beautiful woman—and they wanted their daughter to grow up not simply looking as normal as possible but beautiful. I didn't blame them for this desire; it didn't seem to be shallow or to place too much emphasis on facial beauty. It was a parental desire I would have shared if Ashley had been my daughter or granddaughter. In cases like hers, I could always see possibilities for refinement and would always consider little improvements. As a plastic surgeon who focused on reconstructive work but had been trained as an aesthetic surgeon as well, it was impossible for me *not* to want to give every patient a face that was balanced and harmonious—in a word, beautiful.

Ashley returned to see me on a regular basis, as most of my patients did, and when she was fully grown I did a final secondary lip and nose procedure, and I was delighted—not only by how she looked but by the self-confidence this young woman possessed, the pride she took in her capabilities, and the wonderful compassion she had for others. We had the opportunity during that time to talk and reflect on the journey we had shared, and I came away all the more pleased to have been able to help her become an adult possessed of such talent and insight and grace.

She had attended the University of Texas, where she had been a business major. But before she graduated she somehow knew that her true interest lay elsewhere. She had discovered that she wanted to be a physician, she told me, something I'd heard from other patients, of course, and

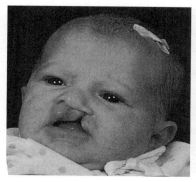

Ashley Ashcroft presurgery infant photo

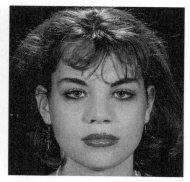

Ashley postsurgery adult photo

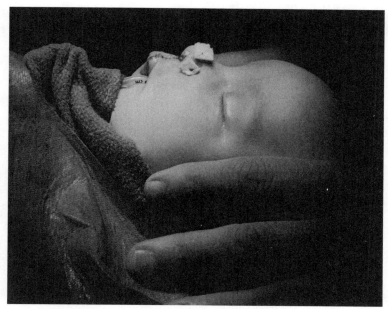

Ashley following correction of her cleft lip and nose

news I couldn't help being happy about, and perhaps a little flattered.

We reminisced about her many procedures and she laughed, recalling that they were "all about Ashley. Before the surgery, I'd get to go shopping and out to dinner somewhere I really liked. Then afterwards, people would send me special things, like cookie bouquets. I'd get to eat red Jell-O for days and days, and all my friends would come over to visit. Even though I did have to have surgery, I always tried to keep a positive attitude. It got me through everything. I concentrated on the good things—seeing my favorite movies, cuddling with my most beloved stuffed animals, and sleeping on special sheets."

Ashley laughed again, then wanted to ask me something as another memory flashed.

"I remember that surgery when I was in the fifth grade—it was a big reconstruction where you did a lot with my nose. I had these giant things in my nostrils that I called 'bright orange trumpets.' What were those things? When you finally took them out it seemed like they were a foot long. I thought you were never going to stop pulling everything out!"

I laughed, too, then explained that the "trumpets" were nasal tubes we placed to provide internal support for her new nose and to press the mucous lining against the septal cartilage, adding that if she did become a doctor, she'd soon know more than perhaps she'd ever wanted to about stents and shunts and tubes of every kind.

Soon thereafter, Ashley did become a premed major, and later was accepted at the University of Texas School of Medicine at San Antonio. Two weeks before the start of classes, however, she made a decision I both understood and supported, in part because my granddaughter, also named Ashley, had made the same one. As much as my patient Ashley was committed to helping people by going into medicine, she was also eager to start a family and become the mother her mom had been. And she worried that six or eight or ten years of intense study and sacrifice would prevent her from having the personal life she wanted.

She shifted her focus and applied to physician's assistant school, and after only three years of training, she had a job she loved that also allowed her to pursue another dream and marry. Today, she works as a PA in the ophthalmology section at MD Anderson Cancer Center in Houston, one of the world's foremost cancer treatment hospitals. It's a great setting, in which Ashley plays a vital role in patient care, and I'm certain that her rapport with her patients is wonderful.

Over the years, I've had many patients who wanted to be surgeons, anesthesiologists, orthodontists, or doctors of some kind. There's no question that their early experiences with the medical world—familiarities they certainly didn't ask for—not only exposed them to a profession that can be fascinating but also formed within them a compassion for others that is invaluable. For many, that profound empathy with the plights of others touches something deep in their souls and initiates their medical careers as an almost mystical calling—and Ashley is one of those, someone for whom work is service, and service is a spiritual practice.

When I recently spoke with Ashley, she reported that when she looks in the mirror these days, she *loves* the face she sees. And she's curiously grateful both to have been born with cleft lip and palate and to have been reconstructed. "It's definitely shaped my personality and beliefs," she explains. "I think being around doctors, hospitals, and other craniofacial patients so much just made me want to give back and help. Even though I'm not working with craniofacial patients now, because of my own experiences I'm able to be more empathetic with *my* patients, who are dealing with all the fear and uncertainty of cancer. I know what those fears are like. I know how much they want to be whole, and what a blessing simply being normal becomes."

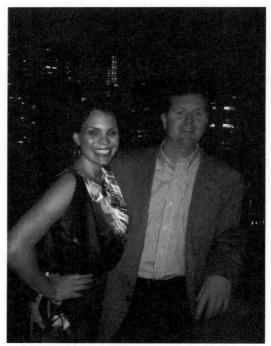

Ashley Ashcroft with her husband

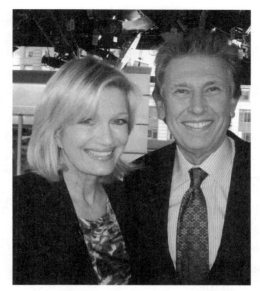

Dr. Salyer with Diane Sawyer

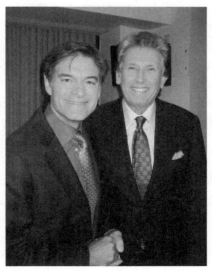

Dr. Salyer with Dr. Oz

Chapter Eleven

Beautiful Faces

An envelope arrived at the World Craniofacial Foundation offices, addressed to me. Inside was a four-page printed document entitled "My Testimony, My Life." And as soon as I began to read, memories of a special patient flooded back to me:

My name is Martin Oliva-Torres. I was born in Guatemala, Central America, on November 5, 1960. I don't know the details, but my mother died when I was three months old. My grandmother took me in to raise. From the beginning that I can remember, grandmother made me believe that I was the reason for my mother's death. So she would beat me every day for no reason. Not only did I feel guilty, but I also had been born with a facial deformity. I was made to be thought of as a monster. Not only was I treated this way by my family, but by everyone. This caused such low self-esteem of myself. I couldn't even hold my head up. I was never allowed to go to school, and it was very hard to find work. Because whenever people would see my face, they wouldn't hire me. This caused me to start drinking at the age of twelve. I thought this would take away the hurt and kill the pain.

I certainly remembered Martin and the surgeries I had performed on him roughly twenty years before. But I had never heard this story—and I was fascinated to continue reading.

When I was about twenty-three, I met a man named Harold. He washed cars so he let me help. One Sunday this American lady came by and asked me to keep an eye on her car. When she returned she asked me if I had seen a doctor. I said why I'm not sick. She said about your face. I told her I didn't have money for

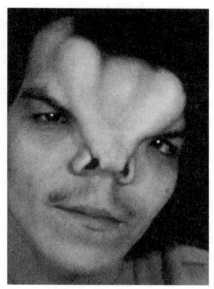

Martin Oliva-Torres

those kinds of doctors. She said in America there are doctors that will do the surgery for free. She gave me her business card and asked me to come to her office the next day. The next Sunday she was back and asked me why I didn't come to her office. I just said I don't know. So she gave me a little money and said come see me tomorrow because very soon we will be taking some children to America for surgeries. She told me her name was Angie.

I did go to the address she gave me and I found that the place where she worked was an orphanage for disfigured children. There were children there with all kinds of deformities. I had always thought no one else looked like me. When I saw all these children the words came back to me that I had heard many years before, "YOUR LIFE IS GOING TO CHANGE." This is when I started calling Angie "my Angel." To this day I can't remember her last name and I haven't been able to locate her to thank her and let her know how my life has changed.

Angie had arranged for my passport. She already had my visa. The next day we were taken by bus to the airport. I was handed a fourteen month old little boy. He was all bundled up in a blanket. They gave me one bottle of milk and no diapers. It was a plane filled with disfigured children. I had no idea what to do. I had nothing, no money, couldn't speak English. I had never been anywhere in my life. When we landed, we were in Houston. They took me and the baby, Bernie, and another little boy, Rolando, off the plane. Our fares only went as far as Houston. We were basically abandoned. *The baby was crying, wet, hungry, had a fever and was covered with chicken pox. I didn't know what to do. One of the ladies at the airport helped me. She was able to get the baby a bottle of milk and clean diapers.*

Somehow they were able to get in touch with a pastor in Arlington to see if he could locate a family to take us into their home. He called everyone in his congregation. He finally found a family to take us, Phyllis and Zane Jude. Phyllis was somehow able to get in touch with doctors to perform the surgeries on the boys. Bernie had a facial deformity and Rolando was born without ears.

This is where Dr. Salyer came into my life. He performed surgery on Bernie and me and I kept hearing, "YOUR LIFE IS GOING TO CHANGE." I really don't know the details of how it came about for my surgery, but he finally made me acceptable to society. So I taught myself English by placing an English and Spanish Bible side by side. Then I was able to get a work permit.

For years I had lost contact with Dr. Salyer. I had gotten married in 2006. Six months after we were married, God called me into his ministry to reach out to others that are hurting. One day my wife Delores and I were watching Oprah and I saw Dr. Salyer there with the Egyptian twins that had been connected at the skull. I couldn't believe it. I didn't know his name or how to contact him before that. When I wrote him a letter, Dr. Salyer called me and wanted me to tell him all about my life since my surgeries. So we made an appointment to visit him in his office. What a reunion that was I will never forget. There were lots of tears and laughter those couple of hours.

If you are not familiar with Dr. Salyer he is the founder and the president of the World Craniofacial Foundation. He has performed surgeries all over the world changing the lives of thousands. I have so much to be thankful for. First I have to thank God my personal savior and for that small voice I kept hearing over and over, "YOUR LIFE IS GOING TO CHANGE." And also for him sending my angel, Angie, who directed me to this world famous surgeon Dr. Kenneth Salyer, who transformed my life for nothing. He transformed me physically and my God transformed me spiritually and mentally. If I ever get the opportunity to write a book, I think I'll title it, THE TOUCH OF THE MASTERS' HANDS: GOD AND DR. SALYER.

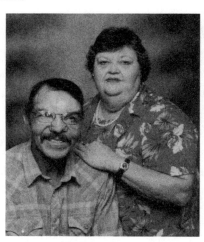

Martin and Delores years after his surgery

When I first met Martin as a twenty-five-year-old, he presented with frontonasal dysplasia, which had resulted in hypertelorism and caused severe disfigurement of his nose, face, and forehead. The distance between his eyes was double what it should have been, and his forehead undulated with wildly abnormal dips and peaks that I had never seen before. Martin offered me a major challenge, but I was excited to try to help. Martin and Bernie had been brought in by their unofficial foster parents, Phyllis and Zane Jude, who simply explained that they were "sort of missionaries" and that the two boys had no one else in the world to look after them.

Bernie had a large protrusion of his brain, known as an encephalocele, coming out from a hole in the bone between his eyes. In a single five-hour operation, pediatric neurosurgeon Maurie Saunders and I performed an intracranial correction, keeping as much functional brain tissue intact as possible, then using split cranial bone from Bernie's skull to create the medial orbital wall and a nicely proportioned nose and forehead for him. And I have to boast that it was one of my true surgical triumphs. A few years later, when Bernie wore glasses, which he needed to correct his vision, it was difficult to see *any* residual deformity, and he looked like an absolutely normal boy.

Soon after the surgery to correct Bernie's encephalocele, I did the first of Martin's several surgeries, a bifrontal craniotomy and bilateral box osteotomies, removing twenty millimeters of bone and the ethmoid sinuses in the interorbital space—just as I had done with Michael Hatfield—and entirely rebuilt his forehead, as I had with Bernie. I created a new nose with the help of excess skin from Martin's

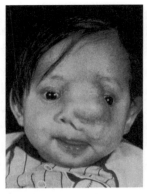
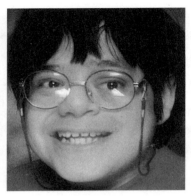

Bernie preoperation   *Bernie ten years after his surgery*

forehead, using the technique called V-to-Y advancement, and the surgery gave him a dramatic improvement.

Martin needed a couple of smaller procedures, and the Judes helped make sure that this determined young man, whom they had literally taken in off the street, made it to all his appointments and closely followed our postoperative instructions. At the time of the surgeries, Martin hadn't taught himself English yet; we could only communicate with our eyes, and I knew nothing about the journey that had led him to me.

When I invited Martin to my office years later—as he described—he was married and working as a school custodian in addition to pursuing his ministry, and it moved me to see how very happy he was with himself and his life. He told me that day about the voice that kept telling him, "Your life is going to change," but until I received his written "testimony," I had never known how easy it would have been for Martin's life to be entirely lost in the alleys of Guatemala City.

I don't believe that things happen by chance. Instead, I think an orchestration of what I call synchrodestiny led Martin and Bernie from Guatemala to me so I could help them lead lives that mattered—to themselves and to the people they encountered. Being able to see the outcome of cases like theirs engenders real joy in me, and it's difficult for me to express how much it means to have had an important hand in saving so many individual lives that otherwise would have been lost.

Once Martin was no longer an outcast and was blessed to experience love and concern from wonderful people like the Judes, his life was transformed. He became spiritually aware and started preaching whenever he was given the chance, spreading the word of God and the importance of faith and belief. In the end, Martin touched me in ways as significant as those in which I touched him, and that small voice also might have whispered to him, "You are going to change other people's lives"—because he has.

I've observed for nearly fifty years how people with facial differences so often have spiritual messages for all of us about what is important—if we will listen. In my experience, regardless of how normal their skulls, foreheads, eyes, and jaws ultimately become, they all have beautiful faces, countenances that demonstrate that love and compassion for ourselves and those around us matter more than anything else. I've said repeatedly over the years that one of my jobs has been to help take my patients "out of the darkness into the light." Now, as my career nears its end, I realize far more clearly than I ever have before how dramatically *they* have taken *me* into a light that shows me truly who I am and why I am here.

*   *   *

By 2006, my peripheral neuropathy largely remained unchanged. It was a nuisance—I couldn't stand the sensation of a sock on the skin of my right foot, for example—but it had never progressed to the point where muscles were weak in either of my feet, or in my legs, arms, or hands. I was blessed by that, and—just as had happened when I was a young boy—I'd faced a difficult medical situation of my own and had dealt with it without having to surrender to it. I turned seventy that year—but seventy is the new sixty, don't they say?—and my fine motor control remained undiminished by time. I was still a good surgeon, and my experience was matched by only a few other surgeons in the world—each of them dear friends—and I had much that I still wanted to accomplish.

Five years before, however, I had committed to the sale of my practice, and the terms of the sale were that I would leave after a five-year transition period. I had hoped that David Genecov, my partner and buyer, would want me to remain part of his team indefinitely, but he was eager to put his own personal stamp on the practice, to shape it in ways of his choosing. David was committed to craniofacial surgery, as was Raul Barceló, but cosmetic surgery was becoming an increasingly significant part of their practice, and perhaps I no longer fit.

Remaining in Dallas for so many years—making it my home in ways this Kansan could never have imagined in his youth—had offered me many pleasures, and one of them was the opportunity to stay in at least occasional touch with patients like Martin, patients who had grown up to make great contributions in all walks of life. Because so many of them required repeated surgeries, I literally watched hundreds of these kids grow up, and for many of them, I joined their parents in being the most important adult in their lives.

Very few of them actually *liked* having to come see me as often as they did, but at the same time, they tended to trust what I told them—that not only could I improve their facial appearance and with it their self-esteem but, when needed, I could also help them breathe, speak normally, see, and hear. It was enormously gratifying to see these young people come into their own as human beings. They came to me as seeds, and I watched them grow and blossom during the years of their surgeries. What a joy it was to see how those blossoms had matured into fruit in the early years of their adult lives.

I saw it with patients like Georgette Couvall, dedicated to helping others with craniofacial abnormalities; with patients like Michael Hatfield, determined to make certain that people with deformities are treated fairly in society; I saw it when someone like Martin triumphed; and I saw it demonstrated once again in the letter I received just the other day from Lacie Carpenter, a lovely Texas girl—now a woman—who was born with a bilateral cleft lip.

"Yes, Dr. Salyer, you're right," she wrote,

> ...*some blessings are disguised as challenges. But those are what make us stronger. For twenty-five years, my life has been full of blessings. Yes, many of them came disguised, but they later transformed....I was blessed with an amazing mother who never accepted anything but my best. I was also blessed by having you and your incredible team. You transformed me on the outside, which strengthened who I am on the inside.*

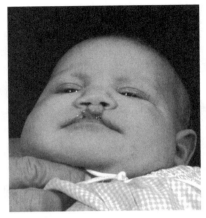

Lacie Carpenter as a baby, preoperation

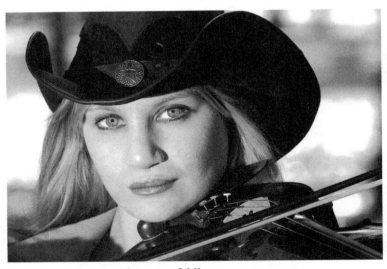

Lacie Carpenter as a champion fiddler

Yes, you and I are both somewhat "strong willed." I always knew we would get along. The physicians and the hospital personnel and my mother helped me grow strong, grounded, determined to succeed, and love life.

The arts have been my outlet for twenty years. Playing my violin/fiddle, acting, singing, and writing have been my way of letting everything out in a healthy, positive way. Music has been my constant.... Making people feel the way I do while I'm performing has been my goal for many years. That is why I decided to major in music education with a specialization in violin performance....

My years in college went quickly by, and as my music transformed, so did I. I became the world champion fiddler and a first-prize fiddler—while still playing in the Orchestra of the Pines Symphony. I performed in Germany, Austria, and London—yet another transformation. My recitals, or as I called them, concerts, went by in a flash. Graduation came—and it was over.... I told you my life has been full of blessings. I also believe that I never meet anyone by accident.

Spring 2012, I was asked to be the featured fiddler in Ireland with a group of highly talented musicians. As the journey began, all I wanted to do was perform and one day become a music therapist. But during my stay my thoughts became clear—medical school—psychiatry. I knew what I had to do first—board certification in music therapy—then on to medical school. I want to do more than teach, I want to do more than to make people feel the way I do about music; I want to help others the way my doctors helped me.

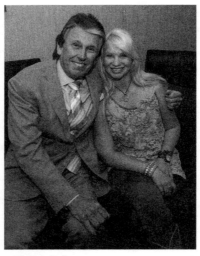

Lacie Carpenter with Dr. Salyer

When I sold my practice, I worried a bit that I would lose contact with people like Lacie, former patients whose rich lives and accomplishments were somehow continuing rewards for my own endeavors—proof that my work was work that mattered. But that didn't happen. I continued to hear from *lots* of them, often when something significant had just occurred—when they had married or given birth to a child—and sometimes, as was the case with Lacie, when they had made an important decision that seemed exactly right for them, one they wanted to share.

I had made a momentous decision of my own that led to my departure from my practice, and although I hated to be surrendering a daily schedule that had invigorated me for forty years, in a number of ways it was exactly the right time to leave. There now were several craniofacial surgeons practicing at Medical City Dallas and elsewhere in the city, and many throughout the United States and the world. But the International Craniofacial Institute, with its stellar interdisciplinary team, its unique academic program, and its vital research division, was gone.

For twenty years, we had created and brought life to a unique center that offered the best craniofacial care in the world. Yet now the clinical and surgical practice that had been headed by Derek Bruce, Ian Munro, and me—and with the mentoring and training that had been so vital to everything we did—carried on in other settings as far-flung as India and Indianapolis, Tripoli and Tampa, Shanghai and Manila and New York City.

I had always been a strong believer in the idea that the best way to help the largest numbers of children with head and facial deformities was to train surgeons and establish centers as broadly across the globe as possible. And that was happening as a new generation of surgeons—trained by those of us who were inspired and mentored by Paul Tessier in Paris—returned to their home countries to work, and also set out to new lands to establish their practices.

That was plenty of legacy for me, and as I continued to lead the World Craniofacial Foundation and to actively consult and perform surgeries in settings around the world, I remained gratifyingly connected to the work Tessier had initiated forty years before when he so determinedly demonstrated to six young surgeons the exciting possibilities of this new approach to reconstructive surgery of the head and face. Ian Jackson, Daniel Marchac, Ian Munro, Fernando Ortiz Monasterio, Linton Whitaker, and I watched and listened, experimented and learned, practiced and practiced some more, then became mentors ourselves of this wonderful, sometimes magical, and almost always transformational surgical subspecialty. And now our students—fine, dedicated surgeons themselves—were at work in operating suites on every continent.

After forty years during which I'd maintained a demanding surgical schedule every week, it was odd at first—and more than a little disconcerting—to don my surgical scrubs so seldom. But the upside was that at long last I could devote attention to the World Craniofacial Foundation in ways that I hoped would lead to the establishment of at least one excellently staffed and operated craniofacial center in virtually every country, regardless of the nation's size or wealth. It was an ambitious goal, but I'd accomplished improbable things before, and the need was great.

The stark reality remained that the vast majority of disfigured children in developing countries still do not have access to the care they need. There simply aren't enough caregivers and facilities to make that possible. A number of organizations and individuals do extraordinary work, but even in the area of cleft lips and palates alone, even if every child born with that deformity could be identified, there still are not enough resources and personnel to successfully treat them. When you consider the full spectrum of craniofacial disorders and their numbers, the task is daunting, but I continue to believe that one day it can be completed.

The work of the WCF is, first and foremost, to identify children with craniofacial abnormalities no matter where they reside and provide them with access to excellent, transformative care offered by a dedicated team of medical professionals. In order to be successful in this mission, it's imperative to broadly educate physicians, surgeons, and supporting staff about the disorders themselves and the state-of-the-art procedures and techniques that can correct them. It's essential to demonstrate that a comprehensive team approach to evaluation, diagnosis, and treatment is not only desirable but fundamental to success—particularly when the goal is reaching out to and treating four hundred or more children over the course of a year rather than only four or five.

Educational programs are extremely important, too: international fellowships, postgraduate surgical fellowships in craniofacial surgery, and visiting professorships all help ensure that knowledge is disseminated broadly and that breakthroughs and advances are quickly and widely shared.

Equal in importance to the creation of excellent centers and the training of their staffs is patient support, ranging from direct financial assistance for families of affected children to a broad range of public information and outreach endeavors. Particularly in developing countries, for example, patients and their families often need assistance in negotiating the clerical requirements that lead to treatment. And if patients don't get to the centers, they can't be treated; something as basic as the cost of a hundred-mile bus ticket to reach a center can make care impossible, even when it is otherwise free.

In many countries, the challenge is not only to provide life-altering treatment to the children who need it but also to influence attitudes toward people with deformities and to increase awareness that *everyone* deserves an acceptable face that functions as it should. Normal speech, vision, and hearing are essential for children's early years, to become the foundations of productive lives, and many permanent disabilities can be prevented with proper early diagnosis and treatment.

The general public must be strongly encouraged *never* to simply lock a child away because of societal fears or the risk of ridicule or embarrassment—or to be the instigators of prejudice themselves. Young adults in their childbearing years need to learn that proper prenatal care improves the chances of giving birth to a normal child. Good nutrition is vital, and something as basic as ensuring that expectant mothers get enough folic acid in their diet can prevent the development of in utero deformities. It's critical, of course, for pregnant women not to smoke or drink alcohol during their pregnancies, but even this information is unknown in many parts of the world.

As I began to devote virtually all of my attention to the foundation and its mission, I was struck by the immensity of the challenge. It was something I had always understood to some degree, yes, but the problems the foundation was organized to meet were global, they were entrenched, and overcoming them demanded both highly technical expertise and significant and sustained funding. I was energized by the scope of the undertaking and by the knowledge of what fulfilling it would mean to hundreds of thousands of children, but I was sometimes daunted—as individuals and groups often are—by the fact that the foundation was a small one and that so much remained to be done. Yet we were not alone.

As long ago as the late 1970s, I had traveled to Taipei, the capital of Taiwan, at the invitation of Dr. Sam Noordhoff, an American plastic surgeon and wonderfully dedicated medical missionary who had moved to that country twenty years earlier. In 1959, he had become the superintendent of Mackay Memorial Hospital, and during his tenure there and then at Chang Gung Memorial Hospital, he had founded centers focused on polio rehabilitation, cleft lip and palate treatment, burn treatment, and suicide prevention. By the time he reached out to me, Sam had become a citizen of Taiwan and was revered nationally as Luo Huei-fu, "Man of Wisdom."

My entire surgical team traveled with me to Taipei in 1978, including a fine pediatric anesthesiologist named Michael Ramsay from Baylor University Medical Center in Dallas; Donnell Johns, a speech pathologist working in the division of plastic surgery at UT Southwestern; plus my stalwart colleagues Ed Genecov, ENT surgeon Trevor Mayberry, and the irrepressible Rosalyn Patterson. We had done very little international travel back then, and the sojourn in Taiwan was a terrific, eye-opening experience, both with regard to the great need for high-quality care in Asia and many other parts of the world and because of our discovery of the impressive facility and team of surgeons Sam Noordhoff already had put together.

With the very generous support of billionaire Y. C. Wang, chairman of the board of Formosa Plastics Corporation, one of the largest plastics manufacturers in the world, Sam was developing a multidisciplinary center whose mission would go beyond the cleft lip and palate repair that had been his earlier focus to include a wide range of head and face disorders whose treatment was just beginning to be known as craniofacial surgery.

With Mr. Wang's funding, we were able to travel with a hundred thousand dollars in US-made surgical equipment.

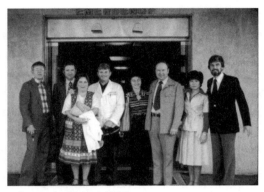

Dr. Salyer and team in Taipei 1978

We were able to demonstrate its use in a number of head and face surgeries during our stay, and, of course, it remained behind after we departed to be used by Sam and his two protégés, Yu-Ray Chen and Fu-Chan Wei, both of whom were young and gifted. Ray, in fact, would become my first fellow in craniofacial surgery soon after I left my position at the University of Texas Southwestern Medical School, then would return to Taipei to direct the craniofacial center at Chang Gung Memorial Hospital after Sam's retirement.

Our initial trip launched craniofacial surgery in Taipei, but the hospital Sam and his colleagues established on the heels of our visit thrived because of their enormous dedication to their work. Sam believed as passionately as I did in a multidisciplinary model for providing service, with neurosurgeons, microsurgeons, orthodontists, and craniofacial surgeons working in concert to provide comprehensive care. It was a model that proved its value; it began to be initiated in other sites around the world, and by the time we were establishing the craniofacial institute in Dallas in the mid-1980s, Sam and his colleagues were developing such a stellar reputation that gifted young reconstructive surgeons from the US, Canada, and Europe were eager to spend fellowship years in Taipei so they could learn from some of the best people at work in the world.

At the same time that Sam Noordhoff was moving the subspecialty dramatically forward in Taiwan, Fernando Ortiz Monasterio, who died in 2012, was also proving in Mexico City that craniofacial centers could do more than thrive in developing countries—they could lead the world in innovation and quality of care.

Only about a decade after I first met Fernando in Paris in 1972 and was dazzled by his personality, his joie de vivre, and his surgical daring and skill, he had become by many accounts the most renowned plastic surgeon in the world. I suspect Fernando has never once gone without his trademark thick moustache in all the years since he's been able to grow one, but it's his electric smile and captivating

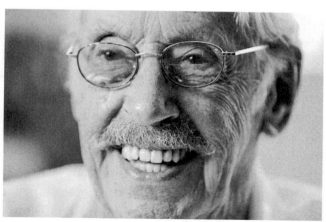

Dr. Fernando Ortiz Monasterio, 1923–2012

personality—together with his extraordinary expertise—that have made him a legend.

He has served as head of the plastic and reconstructive surgery unit of the Hospital General Dr. Manuel Gea González, general director of the hospital, and professor of plastic and reconstructive surgery in the postgraduate division of the medical school of the Universidad Nacional Autónoma de México. He's the author of more than two hundred scientific papers and seven books; he is the only person who is not a US citizen ever to be invited to serve as president of the American Association of Plastic Surgeons, and in 2010, the Universidad Nacional Autónoma de México, his alma mater, awarded him a doctoral degree honoris causa, one of the highest honors bestowed in Mexico.

More importantly still, Fernando created one of the most remarkable craniofacial centers in the world beginning in the early 1980s in a government-funded public hospital whose patients are among the country's very poorest. In Mexico—where a national health-care system has been in place since 1943—overall costs are roughly *one-sixth* of those in the United States, and stellar professionals like Fernando have ensured over the years that the quality of patient care is on par with the best in the world. Yet regardless of the setting or the system, the great challenge remains the same: striving to make a difference with one patient—and one precious life—at a time.

As those centers in Mexico City and Taipei developed and grew, we established vital relationships with them at the institute in Dallas, sharing information and new techniques, incorporating mentoring programs and fellowships that enabled surgeons to spend extended periods at partner institutions, and expanding the horizons for all of us—ever increasing our confidence that we could succeed with procedures that would have been unthinkable even a few years before, and, as always, transforming lives.

In the years since my 2006 departure from active practice, my focus at the World Craniofacial Foundation has been the continual development of centers like those in Taipei and Mexico City and elsewhere around the world, and it's hugely gratifying to me that as I write, the WCF is associated with eleven craniofacial centers in the United States—in New Haven, New York, Cleveland, Cincinnati, Chicago, Indianapolis, Lexington, Winston-Salem, Tampa, Phoenix, and Dallas—and *ten more* centers around the world. The centers in Taipei and Mexico City remain world renowned and show every sign of thriving long after their now-elderly founders have departed. And the WCF also directly provides funding, patient support, professional training, and expertise to centers in Hangzhou and Shanghai in China; Chandigarh, Chennai, and Lucknow in India; Tripoli, Manila, Buenos Aires, and Paris—where my dear friend and recently deceased colleague Daniel Marchac and his partner Dominique Renier worked—and where Eric Arnaud and Alexandre Marchac now continue their work in the city where it all began.

I don't get to perform surgeries as often as I once did, of course. I'm in the operating room only several times a year now instead of several times a week, but the pleasures and the rewards—quite honestly—are almost as great. I visit each of the centers regularly; in person and via telephone and email, I discuss complicated cases with surgeons at each center; I coordinate those instances, for example, in which my Japanese colleague and former fellow Akira Yamada's

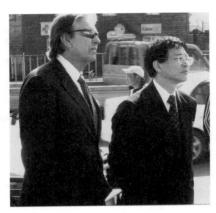

Dr. Salyer in Mongolia

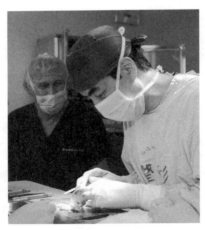

Dr. Akira Yamada, WCF visiting professor

expertise is needed in Mexico City, and I work toward the development of new centers as well.

A few months ago, I traveled with Nagato Natsume, a maxillofacial surgeon and founder of the Japanese Cleft Palate Foundation, and a delegation of surgeons and students from Japan on a mission to Mongolia, where we and the team who joined us performed surgeries, mentored young surgeons, and preached the craniofacial gospel to Mongolian health officials; and I've only recently returned from similar trips to Qatar and the Seychelles as well. From my office in Dallas, I do my best to ensure that each center receives as much direct support from the foundation and its other funding sources as possible. I screen patients who have reached out to the WCF and endeavor to assess their needs and link them to the center I believe is best positioned to offer them excellent care. Most fundamentally, I work as I have for nearly fifty years to guarantee that children everywhere continue to receive from the hands of surgeons normal faces that allow them to bravely face the world.

When I do get to scrub in these days, it's normally because I've been asked to consult on a particularly complex case, and in 2010 my friend and colleague Michael Sadove in Indianapolis invited me to lend a hand with a patient whose surgery he accurately described in a presurgery press conference as "monumental."

Kaydence Theriault was one of three triplets born in Indianapolis in December 2009. Each of the three had Crouzon's syndrome, their skulls closing prematurely in utero while their brains continued to grow, resulting in dangerous disfigurement of their heads. Kaydence's rapidly growing brain pushed her skull into a shocking and very dangerous cloverleaf shape. Instead of a relatively round skull, Kaydence effectively had three—one that bulged out on top of her head and two others that bulged at the sides. Her skull measured just a few centimeters from front to back, and her condition immediately threatened her young life.

Crouzon's is a genetically inherited disorder, and in addition to her brother and sister, Kaydence's mother suffered from Crouzon's, as did her grandfather. Kaydence's birth mates were far less severely affected than she was; they had already undergone surgery and were doing well. Kaydence's extreme condition necessitated surgery as soon as possible, but it was also essential for her surgeons to have a carefully considered plan in place as they commenced.

Kaydence was certainly the most dramatic Crouzon's patient I'd ever encountered when Michael Sadove contacted me in the spring of 2010. He and pediatric neurosurgeon Ron Young had sought my advice because of my track record in rebuilding the skulls of Crouzon's patients, and as we began to discuss Kaydence's situation and our plan of attack, it was vital that we create 3-D models that we could study extensively to ensure safety, accuracy, and an excellent outcome.

Weeks before I flew to Indianapolis for the surgery, we

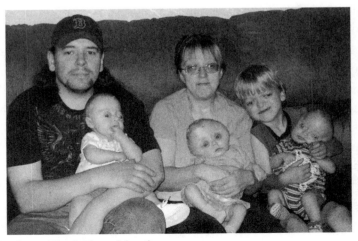

Kaydence Theriault and family

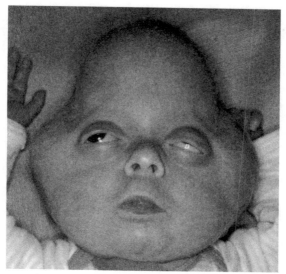

Kaydence presurgery

began to work with Andy Christensen and his team at Medical Modeling in Golden, Colorado. Like both Sam Noordhoff and Fernando Ortiz Monasterio, Andy serves on the WCF board and has offered extraordinary imaging assistance on dozens of complex cases, including the twins Mohamed and Ahmed Ibrahim, and now Kaydence. In videoconferences hosted at his facility, and with physical models in Dallas and Indianapolis as well, we were collectively able to decide how best to sequence and time the procedures we would perform on Kaydence and what specifically we would do.

In Kaydence's brain, the ventricles, which allow the drainage of cerebrospinal fluid, were enlarged to ten times their normal size, and the resulting pressure on her brain was tremendous. With advice from Dr. Derek Bruce—who now lives outside Philadelphia and remains active in retirement as

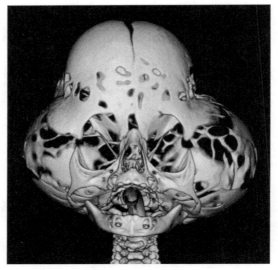

A model of Kaydence's skull prior to surgery

a surgeon consultant for the WCF—Dr. Young had inserted what's known as a functional ventricular peritoneal shunt in hopes that it would decrease the massive expansion of the ventricles and lessen the acute intracranial pressure. The procedure worked, and a few weeks later we were ready to operate.

I had learned many years before that early expansion of the back of the head is the best way to initiate a sequence of surgeries for patients like Kaydence. It quickly lessens the pressure that the skull is placing on the brain, allowing a subsequent surgery on the front of the head, upper face, and eyes to wait till the brain is less traumatized and has had an opportunity to begin to seek its normal shape.

But in Kaydence's case, the severity of her condition meant that several surgeries needed to take place in quick succession, each separated from the others by only a few months. They were three challenging operations, but they all went as well as we had envisioned they would. Each time, Kaydence was in the remarkably good care of anesthesiologist Monty Harrison, and she remained stable throughout surgeries that lasted roughly five hours each.

Her cloverleaf skull was so dramatically misshapen that Ron, Michael, and I needed every trick, idea, and bit of expertise we shared among us to contour her skull into something approximating a normal shape, provide room for her brain to grow and function normally, and ensure as we did so that her brain was never traumatized or injured.

I've mentioned before that in cases like Kaydence's, you never have enough bone with which to work. My preference has always been to use demineralized bone as a second choice when enough of the patient's own bone isn't available. But Kaydence's skull bone was paper thin, and once we had cut it into dozens of pieces, it lacked enough continuity to allow many of the techniques for reconstruction we might otherwise have used. Demineralized bone was not available; the skeletal framework I'd created for Ahmed and Mohamed was not possible; and in the end, we used a synthetic material called Kryptonite that Michael had worked with and liked—and on the heels of three highly intense and complex surgeries, I was delighted with how successful we were.

Kaydence became one of our "WCF kids" along the way, her family receiving direct and indirect support from the foundation, and I know both from that association and from reports by Dr. Sadove that two years after the first surgery, she is doing quite well. Her brain function is entirely normal—she has no cognitive or motor deficits, and she's quickly catching up developmentally with her brother and sister.

I haven't seen her in several months, but in photographs she looks great. She will require more surgery when she's older, once her skull and face have nearly reached their full growth, but the good news for Kaydence—and virtually all Crouzon's patients who receive excellent care—is that by the time she's a young adult, people may never know that once long ago surgeons rather dramatically cut apart and reconstructed her skull, forehead, and face. And that's always our goal.

Each year, more than five hundred cases of children with serious craniofacial disorders are referred to us at the Dallas WCF office. The referrals come from family physicians, surgeons, social workers, and the families of patients themselves, and they come from all around the world. Our goal is to see that each child is treated by the best team and in the most convenient location for his or her particular circumstances. We serve as a triage system, providing expertise, logistics, and support of several kinds during early evaluations, while the children are being treated, and during postoperative recovery and rehabilitation, and we often accomplish it all on a shoestring budget because we're good at soliciting donated and in-kind services for the care of our patients.

Fully ninety-five percent of our annual budget is devoted to program costs, with just five percent allocated for fundraising and administrative costs. I like to think that we're big enough to do the job we've set out to do but small enough to ensure that it's done excellently and that we do indeed

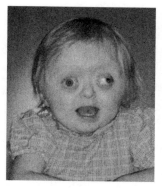

Kaydence after her most recent surgery

meet our mission to give "help, hope, and healing to children and adults with abnormalities of the head and face by providing support and access to life-changing medical procedures."

Sometimes meeting that goal for a single child requires a herculean effort, but that's the point, after all—to do whatever it takes to transform that child's life. As I write, the life of little Grace Kabelenga is very much on my mind. Grace is just such a child, one for whom very daring surgery is absolutely essential if she is to have any kind of life—if, in fact, she is to survive. But her condition is so rare, and surgical reconstruction will be so risky and complex, that her case has already involved surgeons on four continents, the generosity and commitment of resources of national governments and dozens of individuals, and months of detailed coordination between the WCF office in Dallas, craniofacial centers in Argentina and Mexico, and a surgical center in Zambia in southern Africa, her home.

Grace was first referred to the World Craniofacial Foundation in the fall of 2008 by Dr. Goran Jovic, the director of the Interplast Surgical Outreach Center in Lusaka, Zambia's capital. He is the only plastic and reconstructive surgeon in the entire country, where seventy-three percent of the population lives below the poverty level. Because of the severity of Grace's hypertelorism and facial bipartition—which results in part of her brain lying unprotected in the front of her mouth—Dr. Jovic was quickly convinced that she could not be surgically repaired locally when he first examined her a few months after she was born.

As soon as we became involved, we coordinated getting CT scans of her head from Zambia to Colorado, where Andy Christensen and his team at Medical Modeling could create life-size epoxy models of Grace's skull, in addition to sophisticated 3-D images that could be viewed on computer monitors—vital imaging that would allow a number of people scattered around the world to plan a surgery that would be absolutely unique.

Grace, an only child, was born in December 2007 to Elijah Kabelenga, a nursing instructor, and his wife, Ngula, a medical laboratory technician, in Ndola, a city of three hundred seventy-five thousand people, two hundred fifty miles from Lusaka. Grace's condition made it difficult for her to swallow; she was chronically undernourished and anemic but otherwise healthy. Her parents' medical backgrounds made them keenly aware not only of the rarity of her circumstances but also of the enormous effort it would take to successfully treat her. They were devout Christians and assured Dr. Jovic that they could accept what God intended for their daughter, but they were committed to pursuing any avenues that might realistically give her a chance at life.

"I am sure you understand what we have been going

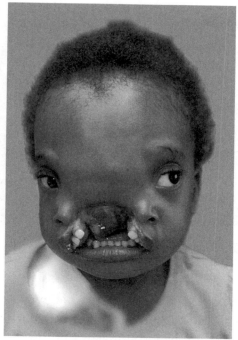

Grace Kabalenga prior to her surgery

through—especially intimidation, stigma, being laughing-stocks, just to mention a few," Elijah wrote in a letter to me. "Had it not been for the grace of God and so much encouraging people like your team, we would be so much devastated by now. We are still trusting God she will one day indeed dance to the glory of God and testify about what God has done for her following her successful operation."

When I began to study the models of Grace's head—endlessly turning them in my hands as I had with so many other challenging cases—it was immediately clear to me that no surgery could be performed for at least a couple

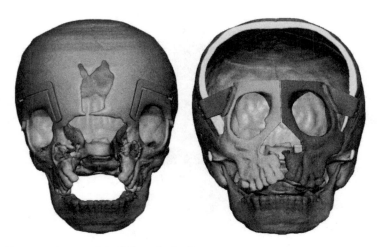

Preoperation model of Grace's skull

of years. Because of the degree to which we would have to reshape the entire skeleton of her face and much of her skull, she would have to grow significantly before that could be accomplished. I knew, too, that her brain's protrusion into her oral cavity would make her reconstruction one of the most difficult I had ever undertaken, yet my heart went out to this little girl, who by all accounts was a delightful and happy child, and I wanted to do everything I could to help her before she died or became self-aware and could understand her plight.

After dozens of consultations over the course of more than two years with Dr. Jovic in Lukasa; my trusted craniofacial colleague Akira Yamada in Japan; my former partner and pediatric neurosurgeon Derek Bruce, now in Pennsylvania; Dr. Martin Chavanne at the craniofacial center in Buenos

Aires; Fernando Ortiz Monasterio in Mexico City; and his successor, Dr. Fernando Molina; and many others, it finally seemed to be the best plan for a team of us from around the world to convene at Hospital Universitario Austral in Buenos Aires in November 2011 for Grace's profoundly complex surgery.

But we suffered a severe setback soon after Grace and her father arrived in Argentina when Dr. Chavanne and his staff discovered in a presurgical workup that Grace was far more malnourished than we'd known, a condition that would make it much harder for her to survive the surgery and would make the postsurgical healing of her wounds almost impossible. We rescheduled her surgery for April 2012, by which time we felt certain that via intravenous feeding and constant medical attention Grace would be in good condition for surgery.

In the following months, Grace was treated for a gastric hernia, which had been aggravating her poor nutrition, and was fitted with a feeding tube. She responded remarkably well, but then another hurdle presented itself. Hospital Austral, which at first had indicated that Grace would receive care as an officially sanctioned charity patient, presented the foundation with a forty-thousand-dollar bill for her treatment to date—just for convalescent care. The costs of her surgery would be in the hundreds of thousands of dollars if the hospital administrators would not relent—and they would not—so we were forced to find another location for the surgery.

I wasn't surprised when Dr. Fernando Molina called not long thereafter to say that he had secured permission from the Mexican national department of health for Grace to be operated on at Mexico City's renowned Hospital Infantil

de México free of charge. He is a gifted craniofacial surgeon, and I have worked so closely with him and his mentor,
Dr. Ortiz Monasterio, over the years that I'd felt sure they
would find a way to help us. Grace and her father traveled
from Buenos Aires to Mexico City at the end of April for a
surgery we planned for early June.

We were five days from the scheduled surgery, however,
when Grace developed an upper-respiratory infection that
once again necessitated postponement. Yet as I write, I'm on
an American Airlines flight from Dallas to Mexico City, and
we will operate on Grace at last in two days' time. Schedul-
ing complications won't allow Akira Yamada to fly in from
Japan, but I'll be joined by my stalwart colleague Derek
Bruce; Dr. Fernando Chico, a pediatric neurosurgeon based
in Mexico City of whom Dr. Molina speaks very highly and
with whom I've been in consultation for several months;
an anesthesiologist on staff at Hospital Infantil; and Jenna
Diaz, who's been my scrub nurse since the time fifteen years
ago when Rosalyn Patterson retired.

Jenna knows my every move and habit and quirk as well
as Rosalyn did, and she's a Spanish speaker, which will
serve us well—and I hope it says something positive about
what it's like to work with me that during the entirety of my
career I've had only *two* scrub nurses. We'll make a great
team, all of us, and we need to, because Grace's surgery will
be a truly momentous one.

Our plan of attack will be to remove the front two-thirds
of her skull in order to extend it and make it larger, to provide room for the brain tissue that now resides far too low in
her skull. Once the skull is removed, we'll be able to lift her
brain out of the sac, which is composed of dura and which

currently protrudes into her mouth, then secure the brain in its proper new position with a large bone graft taken from her cranium.

But with her brain raised, she will have a large hole in her mouth that will have to be sealed to ensure that bacteria cannot enter the brain and cause infection and meningitis—in much the same way that we had to seal Ahmed's and Mohamed's brains against bacterial assault, but at the base of her skull and not at its crown, where it was exposed in the case of the boys.

To close the wide opening, we will have to bring the two halves of her face together, which will require cutting the bony framework away from her skull on each side, then bringing the two together, something like connecting two halves of an eggshell to make it whole again. By cutting the halves loose from their attachment to the skull and rotating them in an arc, we'll be able to secure them in a new and proper position. We'll be able to move the pieces of the entire anatomical puzzle into precise position only because of guides we've created from our 3-D models. Without them, the precision required would be impossible.

Once Grace's skeletal framework has been reconstructed and her brain has been lifted and secured, it will be time to turn to the soft-tissue construction of her nose and nasal passages, her upper lip, and the areas surrounding her eyes. Those procedures will be somewhat akin to what takes place in more conventional cleft surgeries, but at every step we will have to be exceedingly careful to ensure that the hole where her brain previously dropped into her mouth remains sealed, secure, and utterly watertight.

I've been reminded often during the many months of

planning for Grace's imminent surgery of the years of planning that preceded the Ibrahim twins' separation and the reconstruction of their skulls. I've similarly obsessed over the broad plans and minute details of Grace's surgery, been similarly awakened in the night with worry, have similarly resolved with cautious optimism that we can succeed and Grace can thrive—eating and breathing and speaking normally with a face that doesn't frighten others away.

I'm eager to get under way; I'm filled with nervous excitement that I know will give way to a calm and intensive focus as we lift our scalpels thirty-six hours from now. And as the first officer calls from the cockpit to say that our plane is crossing the Rio Grande in Mexico, I realize yet again how very blessed I am. At seventy-five, I'm still physically and mentally able to undertake incredibly sophisticated surgery, still able to step up to enormous challenges and demand the most of myself, just as I did beginning in 1962 and have done in all the years from then until now.

Early in my life, I found my calling and committed myself to a life that would matter—to spending the years allotted to me giving children faces that would allow them to shape lives of their own that would matter as well. How remarkably fortunate I am nearly half a century later and as my life arcs toward its conclusion that, despite all the change and challenge that living entails, that fundamental endeavor remains my focus and my joy.

I say a silent prayer of thanksgiving as the plane cuts through the dusky sky, and I say a prayer of hope for life and grace for Grace.

Seed, Blossom, and Fruit

During the trip Luci, Sue Blackwood, and I made to Africa to celebrate Petero Byakatonda's triumphal return to his village, we also traveled into the far north of Uganda, and into the heart of hell.

With a kind and vastly informative CURE International representative named Sam as our guide, we traveled to Gulu, where we planned to hold a clinic, hoping to meet with some

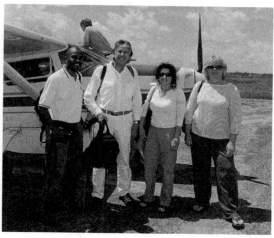

Preparing to fly into Uganda

of the hundred or so "invisible people" whose lives had been all but destroyed by madman Joseph Kony and his so-called Lord's Resistance Army. Since the mid-1980s, Kony and his minions—who claim they are doing God's will—have recruited as many as a hundred thousand children into their wicked cause and have displaced more than a million people in central Africa. Young boys are trained to become killers; girls become the soldiers' prey, and are raped and brutally treated until Kony and his men have no more use for them— but not before many have their ears and noses chopped off and their lips gouged out with knives.

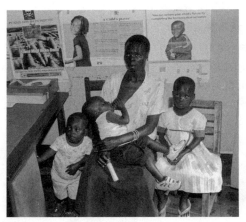

Despair, One of the Invisible People

These young women, most of them now with children of their own, are considered "invisible," people who have been made less than a person via the terrible inhumanity that has visited their lives. I wanted to meet a few of these women, to see if there was any way I could help them, and I'll never forget the first young woman I met. An infant hung at her breast, and a young girl stood close by her side. Both of the woman's ears had been cut off, and most of her nose was gone, too. Yet the truest horror was the vivid evidence that her spirit, her very soul, had been taken as well. Her eyes were vacant, distant, unseeing. She was without expression and almost motionless, as if she were willing herself, as best she could, into a living death where the emotional pain was no longer so severe.

I met dozens more women like her before that terribly sobering day was done, and in the following weeks I met with many people—while we remained in Africa and once we were home again in Texas—hoping to find a way to give these women back a bit of life. But there were so many of them, and the area in which they lived was a war zone, and the cost would have been enormous and the surgical challenges great, so finally I simply had to accept the fact that I could not help. I ached for those horribly abused "invisible people," but I could not help them.

On that same trip, we visited a CURE International hospital deep in the bush outside the city of Mabale. The entire two-million-dollar facility was devoted to the treatment of children suffering from hydrocephalus—swelling of the brain caused by too much accumulation of cerebrospinal fluid—an all-too common problem in underdeveloped regions of the world. The hospital outside Mabale was modern and efficiently run, and it was there, I discovered, that Dr. Benjamin Warf, an American pediatric neurosurgeon, had developed a simple procedure some years before to help children with hydrocephalus. He discovered he could use just a tiny endoscope in a small opening in the skull to dramatically reduce the pressure on his young patients' brains by opening the aqueduct blocking the drainage of spinal fluid in their ventricular system, decompressing the enlarged brain and safely restoring its vital functions.

Elsewhere, the then-state-of-the-art method for treating hydrocephalus still involved inserting a silicone shunt to drain the dilated ventricular system of its spinal fluid. These artificial shunts were prone to become infected over time, however, particularly if the patient lived in primitive or unhygienic conditions. And there in the remote African bush, I was able to scrub and watch one of Warf's African protégés perform a simpler and far better procedure. Today the procedure he pioneered is replicated around the globe, and thousands of children around the world have survived, thanks specifically to his vision and dedication.

I've often considered in the years since that visit to Uganda how stunningly different those two experiences were, and how, within a relatively short reach of miles in a poor African country faced with enormous problems, we had observed the handiwork of humankind at its worst and perhaps its best, too. The contrasts were stunning, and the realities broke my heart and made it soar as well. I've asked myself again and again over the years what, in fact, any of us—or all of us—can do to make the world a marginally better place, or even a far better one for our having lived, and I've gathered a few ideas.

My belief, I'll be honest, is that the very best way to make a difference in the world is to attend fundamentally to ourselves, to care for, nurture, and love ourselves as the starting point for spreading love widely in the world. And because I'm a physician, perhaps it isn't surprising that I think it's vital for us to care for our bodies, to ensure that they are as strong and healthy and vibrant as they can be.

I got lucky; my peripheral neuropathy never worsened in the ways it initially appeared it would. It continues to be an irritant, but not much more than that; and although aging isn't fun, I think we all should focus on making the most of our bodies as long as we need them, understanding that all the wonders of the universe are contained in the limitless number of things of which our brains and bodies are capable. Our bodies give our spirits refuge and they give our spirits wings, and they deserve our love and nurture.

Spiritual leaders around the world are in agreement when they admonish us to live in the present, in this moment, in the time in which we are alive *right now*. The past gave rise to this moment, of course, but the past cannot be adjudicated or somehow set right, and it cannot be relived. And the future is something that inherently never arrives. While we can plan for the future and move toward it, we can only do so in the now. The present moment is all we have, and a key to living well is to fuse all that we are, all that we represent, all that we believe in and work for into the now—because there is nothing else.

It's living in the moment, too, that allows us to be the best we can be. My life has taught me that dedicating yourself to excellence engenders excellence. Visualizing yourself achieving, realizing, accomplishing, triumphing in every endeavor has the power to bring that success into reality—success of every kind. Pay attention to your mistakes and your failures only long enough to learn from them; spring forward from them believing you'll never fail again. Use all the myriad gifts God has given you to transform what you do with your life into a celebration of the gift of being alive.

Work hard. Devote yourself resolutely yet joyously to everything you do. Give everything your all—not because you seek drudgery or because you somehow must pay your dues, but because work is what we were made for. Find true purpose in what you do; bring the calm yet intense focus to it that psychologists call the flow state. Envelop yourself in your undertakings—your job, your play, your relationships—and give them everything you have. We are *homo sapiens*, wise man, yes, but even more fundamentally we are *homo operantes*, working man, and we learn and grow only from what we do. Choose work you love, bring passion to your work, make your work—whatever it is—a spiritual practice, and I promise you that you'll have lived a rich life when your days of work are done.

As I grow older, I'm ever more convinced that what we think about, we become. If we're always fearful, we will be shaped by fear. If we believe that life is hard or unfair, it will be. If we scoff at the truth that each of us creates our own reality, those realities will not be places in which any of us are eager to reside. But if we imagine joy and love and abundance, they will be ours. Trust me. Take control and use your brain, your mind, and your spirit to create the world in which you live.

Then create happiness. Only you can create it, and it comes only from within. If you wait for specific circumstances to make you happy; if you rely on other people to make you happy, or money or fame or position, happiness will seem like a cruel illusion and life will be dreary indeed. When we choose to be happy, when we insist that there is no other state in which we will live, life becomes a blessing and each day is filled with bliss.

Throughout history, the world's major religious traditions have shared a very singular view of how humans ought to interact with one another, and the great prophets and sages have echoed in every era the same remarkably simple creed.

"Such as you wish your neighbor to be to you, such also be to your neighbors," wrote the pagan philosopher Sextus.

"One should not behave toward others in any way that is disagreeable to oneself," reads the ancient Hindu scripture known as the Mahabharata.

"Try your best to treat others as you would be treated, and you will find that this is the shortest way to goodness," suggested the Chinese sage Mencius.

An Islamic scripture known as the Hadith proclaims, "Not one of you is a believer until he loves for his brother what he loves for himself."

And according to the Talmud, in ancient Palestine Rabbi Hillel taught, "What you yourself hate, do not do to your neighbor," only a few decades before Jesus similarly proclaimed, "You shall love your neighbor as yourself."

Has God conveyed this elegant truth to people everywhere? Or have people in all parts of the world discovered a deeply important *human* truth? I'm not sure it ultimately matters. All I know is that I believe with all my heart that serving others, helping them, treating them as you want to be treated, constitutes the most fundamentally valuable and important human endeavor. We are all part of the same human family. Genetically, physically, spiritually, we are all made of the same elements from which the universe was created. When we serve others, we serve ourselves.

I've been blessed to experience this truth firsthand throughout my life, and to share its fruits. In helping challenged children grow and *become*, I've become myself. And I am very grateful.

*　　*　　*

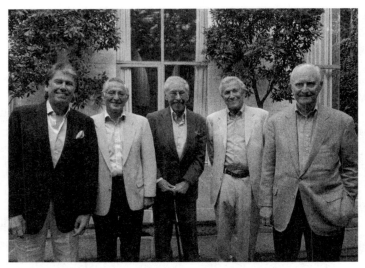

Dr. Salyer with colleagues in Mexico City, June 2012

A couple of months ago, during a time when I was focused on planning the complex surgery for little Grace Kabelenga, I joined four colleagues I've known for forty years in Mexico City. There was no special occasion except our shared realization that we are aging, and we wanted to be sure we all could gather together at least one more time—as we did annually throughout our careers to share our discoveries with each other, to learn and grow and strive together to perfect our craft.

The eldest among us, Fernando Ortiz Monasterio, was about to celebrate his ninetieth birthday, and we chose to rendezvous in Mexico City in part because each of us was very interested in Grace's case, but also because Fernando could no longer travel. Daniel Marchac was still recovering from radiation treatment and chemotherapy but was well enough to join us from Paris; Ian Jackson and Linton Whitaker traveled to Mexico City, too, and we spent three days delighting in one another's company, discussing Grace in some detail as well as other cases, reminiscing about our careers and the surgical subspecialty we had inherited from Paul Tessier and spread throughout the world, and imagining the future.

Fernando described the plans under way for a Mexican team to perform the first full transplant of a patient's face in Latin America at the center he created at Hospital Gea González, surgery that would take place sometime in the coming months. It will be an enormous undertaking, but Fernando's successor, Dr. Fernando Molina, and his protégé Dr. Eric Santamaría, one of the world's most renowned microsurgeons, are very much up to the task. The surgery will follow two highly successful full transplantations of a donor face to a patient recipient in Spain and in France in 2010, one in Boston in 2011, one in Baltimore in 2012, and *three* successful full-face transplantations in Turkey in 2012 as well.

It's certain that face transplants will not become commonplace, but it's wonderful that in the rare instances when they are warranted they will increasingly be available to desperate patients whose own faces have been ravaged by disease or trauma, and those of us who gathered in Mexico City are proud to have spent our careers laying the groundwork that has made full-face transplantations possible. Each of us is too old now to be actively engaged in this new frontier, but we observe it with fascination and more than a little desire to be young enough again to play a role in its development.

Although it's very difficult to accomplish at the moment, I believe that surgeons of the future will be able to create transplanted faces that strongly resemble the appearance of an individual before he or she was beset by the trauma that destroyed an otherwise normal face—something donor families will understand and support. The recipient, after all, is not the donor, whether the gift is a kidney, a heart, or a face.

Facial transplantation will also become an exciting possibility for children and adults with neurofibromatosis, whom we have not been able to help until now. This congenital, progressive disease causes the tumorous overgrowth and often grotesque distortion of the structures of the bones and soft tissues of the head and face. In the past, with excision and reconstruction, we could provide temporary improvement, but the disease normally recurs and progresses—with heartbreaking results. Similarly, many severely burned faces currently cannot be satisfactorily reconstructed, but with increasingly successful face transplantation, those patients, too, will begin to live dramatically renewed lives.

Facial transplantation is made possible, of course, not only by improved craniofacial methods and techniques but also by advances in the parallel field of microsurgery, in which surgeons working with the assistance of high-powered microscopes are able to reconnect tiny blood vessels and repair a wide variety of structures that once were too small and difficult to see, let alone restore or remove. Throughout the world today, microsurgeons can reconnect traumatically amputated fingers and hands and sometimes even entire scalps, in addition to the great advances they have made in transplanting faces.

Perhaps the most exciting area of reconstructive plastic surgery at the moment is tissue engineering. Soon, we will be able to take a patient's own cells and use them to initiate the growth of new tissues that then can be transplanted into the patient to replace organs or body parts lost to disease, trauma, or congenital absence.

I find the nascent developments in tissue engineering thrilling, and they promise an entirely new avenue for the replacement of missing or diseased parts throughout the body. I'm convinced that not too far into the future, tissue engineering will become a commonplace method for surgeons to reconstruct many parts of the head and face. Already in experimental animals, cartilaginous structures like the ear have been grown outside the body, then have been successfully transplanted.

The fundamental building blocks of the body, which were known as precursor cells back when I was in medical school and are commonly called stem cells today, are responsible for the normal continuous regeneration of many parts of our bodies. It's only recently that we've discovered the possibility of harnessing these cells for the creation or stimulation of new tissue and even for the replacement of organs or body parts that have been damaged or destroyed by disease or trauma.

My good friend and fellow plastic surgeon Sydney Coleman in New York, for example, pioneered the use of a patient's own body fat—transplanted at the cellular level—for use in both aesthetic and reconstructive surgery. Although he encountered many naysayers, Sydney is a focused, bright, and inquisitive clinician and researcher, and his innovations proved enormously important to a number of my patients who suffered from Romberg's disease, a rare disorder that causes the virtual melting away of the soft tissues and bones of the face and skull, resulting in large crevices and sometimes major deformities.

Using Sydney's liposculpturing techniques, I've been able to use patients' own fat-derived stem cells to rebuild and recontour their faces, and it's an exciting advance. But Sydney's work has gone even further. He and other people working in the field now have proven experimentally that stem cells derived from a patient's own fat can stimulate the growth of new skull bone—an enormously exciting discovery—and that a number of other body parts and organs can be regenerated from these fat-derived stem cells. I believe it's only a matter of time before the use of stem cells in renewing and regenerating many parts of the body dramatically changes not only plastic and reconstructive surgery but the entire surgical field.

Exciting and very important developments will occur at the genetic and diagnostic levels, too. Today, with the road map for the total human genome in hand, we can diagnose many genetically determined craniofacial diseases and syndromes. Being able to identify the specific gene that is responsible for a given abnormality will almost certainly revolutionize both the treatment and the prevention of craniofacial and other deformities.

New simple, noninvasive blood tests for genetic disorders will undoubtedly decrease the incidence of deformity due to known genetic causes. I've personally observed, for example, how the incidence of simple cleft lip and palate has been markedly reduced in Taiwan by early fetal diagnosis and the subsequent termination of that pregnancy.

Yet with the broad development of genetic diagnosis, it will be vital for societies around the world to develop strict guidelines for the use of abortion as a tool for reducing the incidence of diseases and disorders of many kinds, guidelines that will take into consideration religious and ethical issues, as well as the cost to families and societies to care for diseased and deformed children who come to term. Medicine has always been a field in which scientific advancement and ethical concerns are intricately intertwined. I'm sure that relationship will grow even more profound in the future and that the field of bioethics will become a hugely important one.

There will be a time, I know, when surgeons who follow in our footsteps will look back at the work we did early in the twenty-first century and it will appear rather primitive to them—and that will be as it should be. The advancement of medicine and surgery over the past two hundred years has been a great human achievement. The small role I've played in moving us forward from the early 1960s till now is my legacy, and it's been my attempt to live a life that mattered. What I know most of all is that it's been my privilege and my joy.

It isn't particularly fun for those of us who were Paul Tessier's protégés to be nearing the end of our lives, but that reality is part of the great mystery of living. And there is a profound and comforting truth for me in the fact that the certainty of death is what gives enormous meaning to life.

I'm filled with a sense of the deep rightness of things when I think of the lives of my two children, my six grandchildren, and the generations of children who will follow them—children whose blood will be formed from my blood and whose lives, I trust, will be as etched with purpose and fulfillment as my own.

I think, too, of my thousands of patients and of the way in which they are my offspring of a kind as well. Their rich and good lives have sprung in part from my hands, and their lives honor me. Georgette Couvall is in her midthirties now, and she continues to work tirelessly to assure children with craniofacial abnormalities that their futures are very bright. Luke Rinehart is a ranger in Denali National Park and Preserve in Alaska, living the only life he's ever wanted, one centered on the wonders of the natural world; Lindsey Gozdowski remains stalwart in her plan to become a surgeon. The still-conjoined Dogaru girls are eight years old now and live in Chicago; in school, Tatiana likes mathematics and Anastasia excels in art. At home in Cairo, Ahmed and Mohamed Ibrahim are eleven now and soon will complete elementary school. The boys love soccer and both still speak excellent English and talk often about returning to the United States one day. Jermaine Gardner continues to perform piano concerts around the world; Shawn Coleman, a college graduate now, still works at the Department of the Treasury and reads avidly in Braille. Petero Byakatonda and his family moved from their village five or six years ago, and we are out of touch. But he's a young man by now and perhaps has children of his own. I like to imagine him sitting with a boy and a girl on each knee, offering each one his broad and enveloping smile and teaching them to sing, "God, we have come in front of you. Please bless us and keep us."

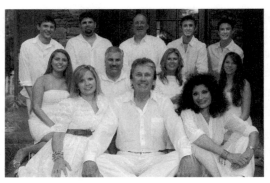

Dr. Salyer with his family

Acknowledgments

This book could never have been written without the many decades of love, support, and guidance offered me by my late father, Everett, and my ninety-eight-year-old mother, Laurene. They set my life on its path and encouraged me to savor the journey, and I am forever grateful.

My deep thanks as well to Sue Blackwood, the executive director of the World Craniofacial Foundation, for the many ways in which she supported the writing of this book, and for her unwavering support of children around the world whom the foundation helps offer new lives.

Mike Lorfing and Marcus Lopez offered many hours of assistance in compiling the photographs that accompany the text. I offer my thanks as well to the Eddie Adams Photographic Archive at the Dolph Briscoe Center for American History at the University of Texas at Austin for permission to reproduce numerous photographs my late friend Eddie made of my patients and me, and to the Sixth Floor Museum at Dealey Plaza for permission to reproduce photographs from President John F. Kennedy's visit to Dallas in November 1963.

Beginning in the spring of 2010, I've worked closely with writer and filmmaker Russell Martin in the creation of this book. During that time, Russell also produced and directed the documentary film *Beautiful Faces*, which chronicles the work of my late dear friend and colleague Dr. Fernando Ortiz Monasterio, whose groundbreaking craniofacial clinic in Mexico City has transformed the lives of thousands of children over the past forty years. I'm grateful to Russell for his creative assistance, for sharing my belief that every child deserves a normal face, and for his friendship.

Kenneth E. Salyer, MD
Dallas, January 2013

About the Author

KENNETH E. SALYER, MD, is a pioneer in craniofacial surgery whose illustrious career has spanned almost half a century. He was the first chairman of the department of plastic surgery at the University of Texas Southwestern Medical School and he established the International Craniofacial Institute and the Cleft Lip and Palate Treatment Center. He has served as president of the International Society of Craniofacial Surgery, American Society of Maxillofacial Surgery, and the American Society of Craniofacial Surgery, and as chairman of the Plastic Surgery Research Council and the American Academy of Pediatrics Section of Plastic Surgery. He is the founder and chairman of the board of the World Craniofacial Foundation. He has published more than two hundred scientific papers and book chapters, and is the author or editor of nine books on craniofacial surgery. He has been a visiting professor at more than fifty medical schools around the world, where he has received numerous honorary memberships, professorships, and degrees. Dr. Salyer lives in Dallas, Texas, and Telluride, Colorado.